Keto Diet Slow Cooker Cookbook 2020

Healthy Delicious Ketogenic Diet Recipes for Rapid Weight Loss, to Optimize Your Health, and Improve Your Life (And to Burn Fat Forever in Just 21 Days)

Jenna Andrews

Table of Contents

INTRODUCTION 1

CHAPTER 1: WHAT IS THE KETOGENIC DIET?.. 2

    ARE THERE DIFFERENT KETOGENIC DIET TYPES? 3

    THE KETO DIET AND WEIGHT LOSS 5

    OTHER HEALTH BENEFITS... 5

    FOODS TO AVOID ON THE KETOGENIC DIET.. 6

    FOODS THAT YOU CAN ENJOY ON THE KETOGENIC DIET 7

CHAPTER 2: WHAT IS THE PROCESS OF KETOSIS AND WHY IS IT IMPORTANT 9

    KETOSIS EXPLAINED 9

    HOW TO ENTER KETOSIS? 10

    WHAT IS THE DIFFERENCE BETWEEN KETOSIS AND KETOACIDOSIS 11

CHAPTER 3: WHAT FOODS CAN I CHOOSE ON THE KETOGENIC DIET?........................... 13

    SEAFOOD 13

    LOW CARB VEGETABLES.. 14

    DAIRY PRODUCTS.. 14

    MEAT AND POULTRY 15

    EGGS 15

    COCONUT AND OLIVE OIL 15

    NUTS AND SEEDS.. 16

    BERRIES 16

    BUTTER AND CREAM 17

    SHIRATAKI NOODLES 17

    UNSWEETENED TEA AND COFFEE 17

    DARK CHOCOLATE 18

    FOODS TO AVOID 18

CHAPTER 4: THE AMAZING HEALTH BENEFITS OF THE KETOGENIC DIET 20

    CAN REDUCE YOUR APPETITE 20

    LOSE MORE FAT IN THE BELLY.. 20

    A DROP IN YOUR TRIGLYCERIDES 21

    CAN REDUCE YOUR INSULIN LEVELS AND YOUR BLOOD SUGAR LEVELS........ 21

    CAN HELP TO LOWER YOUR BLOOD PRESSURE 22

    FIGHTS OFF METABOLIC SYNDROME... 22

    HELPS WITH YOUR LEVELS OF CHOLESTEROL 22

    IT CAN DO SOME WONDERS FOR SEVERAL BRAIN DISORDERS 23

    THE DIET CAN HELP YOU LOSE WEIGHT 24

CHAPTER 5: ARE THERE ANY PRECAUTIONS I SHOULD TAKE WITH THE KETOGENIC DIET? 25

    THE KETO FLU 25

SUGAR CRAVINGS 26

DROWSINESS AND DIZZINESS 26

A REDUCTION IN YOUR STRENGTH AND PHYSICAL PERFORMANCE 26

LOW LIBIDO 27

HOW TO AVOID HYPOGLYCEMIA 27

CHAPTER 6: THE GREAT BENEFITS OF THE SLOW COOKER **29**

KNOWING YOUR SLOW COOKER 30

TIPS AND SAFETY FOR THE SLOW COOKER 30

CHAPTER 7: TIPS FOR FOLLOWING THE KETOGENIC DIET WHILE USING THE SLOW COOKER **33**

DO IT WITH FRIENDS 33

SLOWLY ELIMINATE SOME OF THE CARBS THAT YOU ARE CONSUMING 33

PLAN AHEAD A LITTLE 34

SET GOALS 34

LOOKING AT LABELS 34

WORKOUT WITH THE DIET 35

MAKE A MEAL PLAN 36

CHAPTER 8: YOUR 21 DAY MEAL PLAN FOR FASTER RESULTS **37**

CHAPTER 9: SLOW COOKER EARLY MORNING BREAKFASTS **39**

BACON AND SPICED EGG BAKE 39

CHAPTER 10: SOMETHING ON THE SIDE – EASY SIDE DISHES **56**

GARLIC BRUSSEL'S SPROUTS 56

CHAPTER 11: LUNCHES FOR THE CAVEMAN IN YOU **73**

BEEF MINCE AND SAUSAGE CHILI 73

CHAPTER 12: DINNERS THAT WILL HAVE YOUR FAMILY BEGGING FOR MORE **90**

MEAT LOVER'S PIZZA 90

BEEF AND VEGGIE STEW 98

CHAPTER 13: TASTY DESSERTS **113**

KETO HOT CHOCOLATE 113

Introduction

Congratulations on purchasing *Keto Diet Slow Cooker Cookbook 2020* and thank you for doing so.

The following chapters will discuss more about the ketogenic diet, and some of the basics that you need to know in order to turn this diet plan into your new lifestyle change. Many people have heard about the ketogenic diet in the past, and many people are interested in learning more, understanding how the process works, and even implementing it so they can see the results they want, such as weight loss and improved health, in no time.

This guidebook will start out with information on the ketogenic diet. We will look at some of the basics that come with this diet plan, what ketosis is, the foods that you can eat, and the ones you should avoid, and even some of the health benefits that you can get while on the ketogenic diet that you aren't able to see on other diet plans. We will also have a discussion on things to watch out for on this diet plan and some of the tips you can follow to stick with the ketogenic diet while also using the handy slow cooker.

From here, we will explore the meal plan, along with some of the great recipes, that you can use to see results with the ketogenic diet quickly. Unlike some of the other diet plans you may have tried out in the past, the ketogenic diet makes it easy to lose weight in just a few weeks. We will provide you with a 21-day meal plan, and recipes, to ensure that you are able to lose weight quickly and efficiently.

When you are ready to use the ketogenic diet to lose weight, and you are excited to see some of the results quickly, make sure to take a look at this guidebook and learn more about how to make this diet plan work with the help of the slow cooker.

There are plenty of books on this subject on the market, thanks again for choosing this one! Every effort was made to ensure it is full of as much useful information as possible, please enjoy!

Chapter 1: What is the Ketogenic Diet?

The ketogenic diet, or the keto diet, is a low carb, high fat, and moderate amounts of protein diet that can provide the body with a ton of health benefits. In fact, in a more than 20 studies, it has been shown that this kind od diet can make it easier for you to lose weight and improve your overall health better than any other diet plan out there. Ketogenic diet may even be able to help fight against health issues like Alzheimer's, epilepsy, cancer, and diabetes.

Knowing how the ketogenic diet works, and all of the different parts that come with it, can make it easier for you to learn how to get started with it, and whether or not this is the right type of diet plan for you. Compared to the traditional American diet, and other diet plans that you may have tried out in the past, the ketogenic diet is going to be a bit different. But overall, you will find that it can do some wonderful things for your health and your life.

When you go on the keto diet, you will need to drastically cut down on the number of carbs that you consume. While the traditional American diet will take in about 200 grams of carbs each day, the keto diet is going to keep you under 50 grams of carbs for the day, and sometimes it will put it down to 20 grams of carbs a day. When this happens, your body will get better at burning fat and using that as energy. It will also turn the fat into ketones in the liver, which then allows it to be used as an energy supply for the brain.

The ketogenic diet realizes that by eating carbs as your primary energy source, you are really putting yourself into a vicious cycle of always needing more fuel and taking in more calories than you need. The body likes using these carbs as fuel because they are easy, but they often come with a price. While you are taking in a lot of calories, the carbs will run out of energy and cause you to crash, making it hard to get off the couch and move around, while still making you hungry and want to eat more. These carbs may be an energy source for your body, but it is not the most efficient method of energy and is causing you a lot of health concerns.

So where are you going to get your energy source if you start to cut out all of the carbs that you already eat in your diet? You still need to have a source of energy to keep the body moving, but where is it going to come from? Basically, with the ketogenic diet you are going to train the body off the carbs and get it to rely on healthy fats as their main energy source.

Healthy fats are a much more efficient form of fuel for the whole body. They are filling so you will not need to eat as many of them as before and you will find that the body is able to burn through this quickly. Once the body has time to go through the fat that you bring into it through your meals, it is going to start working on the stores of fat that are in the body, helping you to lose some of the fat that is all over your body.

While carbs were working against you, causing you to eat more and turning into belly and thigh fat when you weren't able to keep up with it, fat is going to be more efficient for the body to burn through. Even when you eat the amount of calories that you need each day, the body is going to be so efficient at burning through all those calories that you will be able to see all the toning and slimming without feeling deprived.

The overall goal of the ketogenic diet is to make you go through the process of ketosis. This is basically the process of changing the body's fuel source from carbs over to fats. The fewer carbs that you are able to eat during this time, the quicker you will get into ketosis. Once you reach the state, you will still need to keep the carb content low so that you stay in this process and work on burning the fat as quickly as possible.

You will be able to eat some carbs, but you do need to limit how many are in the diet so that you can stay on the process of ketosis. It is best to stick with 5 percent or less of your daily calories coming from carbs. This usually means that a serving or so of vegetables it all you will get during the day, but you will be able to enjoy other foods that contain the nutrients that you need and will fill you up.

The majority of the calories that you will enjoy come from the fat that you should be eating. Up to 75 percent of your calories each day should come from fat sources. You do need to be careful though. Counting saturated fats and fats that you get from processed and fast foods will be bad for the heart and go against what this diet plan is all about. Picking good healthy fats, like those from healthy meats, fish, and butter, can provide you with the energy that you need.

Also, make sure that you are adding in some protein to the diet plan. This is not going to take up as much space in your caloric intake, but it is more than you will get with the carbs. This makes it easier sometimes to get the fat content that you need since many good protein sources can also contain all the extra fat that your body needs in the day.

For those who follow the ketogenic diet for some time, you will find that the body will become really efficient at burning fat for energy in a very quick manner. While the body may be used to utilizing carbs and glucose as its main energy source, this is not always seen as the most efficient manner to work with. But once the body switches to fat, it is able to do a world of good, including reducing blood sugar and insulin levels. This, along with a larger amount of ketones in the body, can have many health benefits.

Are There Different Ketogenic Diet Types?

The ketogenic diet is really nice because it can be modified and adjusted to work well for almost anyone who is looking to see some results with their overall health. There are actually several different versions out there when it comes to the ketogenic diet, which means that it is possible to pick the one that works with your lifestyle and your activity level. The different versions out there for the ketogenic diet includes:

1. The standard ketogenic diet. This is the standard version that we are going to discuss in this guidebook. It is a very low carb, moderate protein, and

high fat diet. Most of those who decide to work with the ketogenic diet will only consume 5 percent of their calories from carbs, twenty percent from protein, and up to 75 percent from fat.

2. Cyclical ketogenic diet. This is the version where you will have periods of refeeding with higher carb content during that time. This means you may spend five days in a row on a low carb diet, and then have that turn into two higher carb days.

3. Targeted ketogenic diet: This is the version where you can make sure that you get your carbs right around your workouts. This one is preferred by some athletes because it ensures that you are taking in the number of carbs that you need to maintain your intense workouts.

4. High protein ketogenic diet: This is going to be similar to what you see with the standard ketogenic diet. But you are going to take in more protein. This version will often include about 35 percent instead of the 20 percent.

However, when it comes to the studies on the ketogenic diet, the high protein and the standard versions are the only ones that have been studied extensively. The targeted and cyclical versions are seen as more advanced methods and primarily used by athletes and bodybuilders. The information that we will talk about the standard ketogenic diet.

Staying on the ketogenic diet doesn't have to be too challenging, it is just a matter of changing around some of the things you are eating and pick options that are healthier for you. Keeping track of the foods that you are allowed to eat with this diet are pretty basic. You will want to concentrate on foods that are high in fats, since 75 percent or more of your daily calories need to come from fat. There are quite a few options that you can choose including fatty meats, butters, creams, and so on.

Next on the list is the protein sources. Unless you are going with a higher protein version, you will probably stay at around 20 percent of your daily calories coming from protein and most of your protein sources will also be really high in the fats that you need, such as fish, ground beef, and various types of nuts. Having a wide variety of options can make all the difference in helping you to eat lots of good foods while getting the protein that the ketogenic diet needs.

And finally, you will be allowed to have some carbs on this diet plan, but you need to lower them as much as possible. The fewer carbs that you are able to consume when starting this diet, the easier it becomes to get into the state of ketosis. This will help you to burn the fat that you want out of your body faster. It is recommended that you stick with 5 percent or less of your daily calories coming from carbs and most of these should come from berries and healthy vegetables so that you get the healthy nutrition that you need.

The Keto Diet and Weight Loss

One of the biggest reasons that people choose to go on the ketogenic diet is because it can help them to lose weight, and will lower their risk factors for many diseases. In fact, there is research that shows how the ketogenic diet could be a much better option for helping with weight loss compared to the common low-fat diet. And since this plan is so filling, you are able to lose the weight that you want, without having to track all the food you eat or without worrying about the calorie counting.

In fact, one of the studies out there found that people who went on the ketogenic diet were able to lose about 2.2 times the weight compared to those who went on a low fat diet that was restricting calories. There were also some improvements to HDL cholesterol and triglyceride levels.

Another study that was done concerning the ketogenic diet was about to find that those who went on this plan lost at least three times more weight compared to those that went on the diet plan that Diabetes UK recommended to patients. All of this comes to show how the ketogenic diet can be just the answer you are looking for when it is time to lose weight.

There are several reasons why the ketogenic diet is seem as the best way to lose weight and feel amazing. One of these is the increased amount of protein that you take in. This alone can provide you with more of the nutrients that you needs. And protein is known to be very filling, which can help you to cut calories and still feel satisfied with the food you are eating.

Other Health Benefits

Even though many people choose to go on a diet plan in order to help them lose weight, the ketogenic diet is about so much more than that. You can actually enjoy a lot of other health benefits in the process as well. Some of the other health benefits that you may enjoy when you are on the ketogenic diet include:

1. Fight off diabetes: Since you are reducing the number of carbs that you take in each day, and you don't have to worry about as many sugars either, you will find that it is much easier for you to fight off diabetes and prediabetes with the ketogenic diet.

2. Acne: Lower levels of insulin, and eating less processed foods and sugar, can help you to see an improvement to the amount of acne that you have.

3. Brain injuries: One study that has been done on animals found that the ketogenic diet is able to reduce the rate of concussions and can make it easier to recover after a brain injury.

4. Polycystic ovary syndrome. Since you are able to reduce the levels of insulin in the body when you are on this diet plan, it is possible that it can play a key role in polycystic ovary syndrome.

5. Parkinson's disease: One study has found that this type of diet plan is able to help improve and maybe even prevent the symptoms that come with Parkinson's disease.

6. Epilepsy: One of the first reasons that the ketogenic diet was developed to help fight off epilepsy in children. And this plan can still be used in order to felt fight off this disorder as well.

7. Alzheimer's disease: The ketogenic diet has been shown to help reduce the symptoms of Alzheimer's disease. And for those who already have this disorder, the ketogenic diet is able to slow the progression.

8. Cancer: Currently, there are several types of cancer that are exploring how the ketogenic diet can help improve the prognosis and even fight off tumor growth.

9. Heart disease: The ketogenic diet is able to help improve a few of the risk factors available for heart disease. This includes issues like body fat, blood sugar levels, blood pressure levels, and HDL cholesterol levels.

Foods to Avoid on the Ketogenic Diet

When you get started with the ketogenic diet, you will find that there are quite a few foods that you will need to avoid in order to see results. You will obviously need to avoid any foods that have a lot of carbs inside them or you will kick the body out of the process of ketosis. Some of the other food types that you need to be careful about when you are working with the ketogenic diet includes:

1. Foods with sugars: This includes options like candy, ice cream, cake, smoothies, fruit, and soda.

2. Grains and starches: This would be any product that is wheat based, such as bread, along with cereal, pasta, and rice.

3. Fruit: You can have a bit of fruit, but for the most part, it needs to be eliminated. Fruit, even though it is considered healthy, does have sugars and carbs inside. If you are going to eat fruit, keep it to smaller portions of berries.

4. Beans and legumes. This would include some options like lentils, chickpeas, kidney beans, and peas.

5. Any products that are considered diet products: These are often going to be processed and they can be higher in carbs as well.

6. Tubers and root vegetables. These are often going to have higher amounts of carbs in them as well. You should avoid some options like parsnips, carrots, and potatoes.

7. Condiments and sauces. Make sure that you are checking the labels. Some of these are going to contain a lot of unhealthy fats and lots of sugars.

8. Unhealthy fats: While fats need to be consumed in higher amounts in the ketogenic diet, you need to make sure you are eating the right kinds. Make sure that you avoid options like mayonnaise and vegetable oils that have been processed.

9. Alcohol: Because they are going to be higher in carbs, it is best to avoid alcoholic beverages to ensure you don't kick yourself out of ketosis.

Foods That You Can Enjoy on the Ketogenic Diet

Now that we have taken a look at the ketogenic diet and some of the foods that you need to avoid when you want to enter into ketosis, it is time to turn it around. We want to take a look at some of the foods that are allowed and encouraged on this diet plan. For this one, you want to remember that all of the foods need to be low carb, moderate protein, and high fat options. Some of the choices that you can make to eat healthy on the ketogenic diet includes:

1. Condiments: There are some seasonings and condiments that you are able to use to add some flavor into your food. You can work with spices, healthy herbs, pepper, and salt and still remain keto.

2. Low-carb veggies: Most vegetables are fine, as long as you make sure that they are low carb. In fact most, if not all, of the carbs that you consume should come from healthy sources of vegetables. Consider some options like tomatoes, peppers, green vegetables, and onions.

3. Healthy oils: This primarily is going to mean avocado oil, coconut oil, and olive oil.

4. Nuts and seeds: You can enjoy these as a nice crust on some of the meats you cook, or take a handful as a snack in the afternoon. Some options that go well include chia seeds, flax seeds, pumpkin seeds, walnuts, and almonds.

5. Cheese: If you are adding some cheese into your meals, make sure that you go with options that are unprocessed.

6. Cream and butter: These are just fine to add into the diet. Just make sure that you look for options that are grass fed.

7. Eggs: Eggs are a great option to work with when you want to make a delicious breakfast. Try to go for options that are omega-3 whole or pastured.

8. Fatty fish: There are so many benefits that can come from adding in some fatty fish to this diet plan. Mackerel, tuna, trout, and salmon can all be great options.

9. Meat: turkey, chicken, bacon, sausage, ham, steak, and red meat are all great ways to get the protein and the fat that you need into your diet plan.

When you are at the grocery store, work to base your diet on single ingredient foods, and make sure that it is whole and healthy. This ensures that you aren't getting any processed ingredients into your diet, and that you will be able to get the best results possible out of this diet plan.

Chapter 2: What is the Process of Ketosis and Why Is It Important

An important part of the ketogenic diet is the process of ketosis. Ketosis is a natural state for the body, when it has stopped burning carbs and it relying on fat instead. This is something that is normal during a fasted state or when you are on a low carb diet like the ketogenic diet.

There are a lot of different benefits that can come from being in ketosis. Often it is seen when you want to lose weight quickly, improve your performance, and even see an improvement in your overall health. But there are some times when being in this state can cause issues, which is why you should be careful when you decide to go on the ketogenic diet. For example, those with type one diabetes, and other rare situations, will find that being in excessive ketosis could be dangerous. Let's take some time to look more in detail about the process of ketosis and how it can work to benefit you when you are in the ketogenic diet.

Ketosis Explained

The keto that comes from the word ketosis is going to come from the word ketones. These ketones are small fuel molecules that are found in the body. This is an alternative fuel for the body that can be produced from the fat we choose to eat, and when we have used up all the glucose, or the blood sugar, that in short supply. These ketones are going to be produced when you eat very few carbs (and these carbs are the main source of blood sugar), and when we only consume moderate amounts of protein (if we eat too much protein, it gets converted into sugar in the body.

Under these circumstances, the liver is going to convert the fat into ketones, and then they are released into the blood stream. They will then be released into the blood stream and used as fuel by the cells of the body, just like what we see with glucose. The brain is even able to use these ketones as a form of energy.

One way to enter into this state of ketosis is to follow the ketogenic diet that we will discuss in this guidebook. Another option is to go on a period of fasting. Under these two circumstances, as soon as the body starts to run out of its glucose stores, the whole body is going to switch to relying on fat as a fuel source. The levels of insulin, the fat storing hormones will go down. This helps to increase the amount of fat burning that occurs in the body.

When all of this happens, you will be able to access the fat stores in the body, and in addition to the fats that you consume, you will be able to burn off the fat stores as well. This can be a great way to lose excess weight. In fact, there are studies that show how those who go on a ketogenic diet will be able to provide a faster rate of weight loss, and other health benefits, compared to some of the other diet plans you may have tried. And since you can follow a low carb or a ketogenic diet for any length of time you want, it can help you to get the results with weight loss, no matter how much you have to lose.

How to Enter Ketosis?

Entering ketosis is going to be easy when you start on the ketogenic diet. In fact, if you are able to lower your carb intake enough, and focus on plenty of healthy fats and moderate amounts of protein consumption, this process is going to begin. So, simply by following the macronutrient requirements that come with the ketogenic diet, you will be able to enter into this process.

When you follow most other diet plans, your body is going to rely on lots of glucose, from the carbs and the sugars that you consume, to fuel it. The body likes using this as a fuel source because it is easy, and doesn't take much work for the cells to use. But, the cells often don't use it very efficiency, and you will end up storing much of this as body fat because the cells aren't able to use it properly.

What makes this even worse is that even though you don't go through and use all of the glucose, the body will still crave more and more. This starts a vicious cycle of eating too many carbs, storing the extra as fat, and gaining weight and lots of health problems in the process.

When it comes to the ketogenic diet, you will be able to stop this process. You will cut out the carbs, only eating very limited amounts of them each day, and replacing them with healthy fats and proteins. When the body isn't able to find the glucose as energy, it will have to start searching around in hopes of finding something else to use as energy. During this time, you are going to feel worn out, tired, and have some headaches and other side effects. This is simply because the body hasn't adjusted and this means you are low on energy.

But the body is adapted to burning fat as a source of energy as well, it just needs the time to do this properly. After a few days for most people, the body will start converting the fat into energy and your energy levels will go higher than ever before. The body is very efficient at burning through the fat that you consume, and you will find that it is possible to burn through all the fat you are consuming along with the fat that is stored up in the body when you go on the ketogenic diet.

But to enter into the process of ketosis, and to actually gain all of the benefits that are promised with this diet plan, you must make sure that your carb content is low enough. There are several testing methods that you can use that will help you know if you are actually releasing ketones and that you are on ketosis. You can then adjust the amount of carbs that you eat to help you get into, and maintain the ketosis that you need for the best results.

What is the Difference Between Ketosis and Ketoacidosis

Now, there are going to be a lot of misconceptions that can show up in concerns with ketosis. But the most important and the most common one is that people often get it mixed up with ketoacidosis, a rare and dangerous medical condition that is usually just going to happen with those who have type 1 diabetes if they don't take their insulin. It is possible that some health care professionals will mix up these two as well, maybe because they don't understand how they work or because the names sound alike, which can make the misconception a bigger issue. But it is important to know that ketoacidosis and ketosis are not the same thing.

Ketosis is a very natural state of the body, and we are able to fully control it. There are two situations where it occurs. Either after a period of fasting, either one you chose to go on or one that happened after a period of illness. It can also happen when you go on a low carb diet. The body can naturally go into ketosis when either of these two situations appear.

On the other hand, ketoacidosis is a severe malfunction of the body. This is going to happen when there is an excessive amount, and an unregulated production of ketones. This is going to lead to some symptoms of stomach pain, vomiting, and nausea and then can be followed by confusion. If it is not taken care of in the proper manner, it can lead to a coma. Ketoacidosis is going to require some urgent medical treatment, and it can end up being fatal.

Most people who follow the ketogenic diet, or another low carb diet plan, are never going to reach above three millimolar or so in terms of ketones. And in fact many will struggle to get above 0.5. If you go for two or more weeks without food, you may end up closer to the 6 range. But when ketoacidosis, you will end up with at least 10, and often above 15, millimolar. So you can see that these numbers are completely different between ketosis and ketoacidosis.

There are three possible situations where ketoacidosis is more common. These will include:

- Type 1 diabetes: This is often the most common situation of getting into this condition, especially if you don't take care of the diabetes. As you body lacks the insulin that is needed, you must go through and inject the amount that you need. Even on the ketogenic diet, you will still need to take in some insulin to prevent this issue.

- Some medications that have SGLT-2 inhibitors. These are usually taken when you are suffering from type 2 diabetes.

- Breastfeeding: In some severe cases, following the ketogenic diet while you are breastfeeding can cause ketoacidosis. This is why you may want to wait until after pregnancy and breastfeeding before starting this kind of diet plan.

Ketoacidosis can cause some illness in the body. You will feel sick, nauseous, and very weak. There is a simple treatment if you feel that this condition is happening. You simply need to ingest some carbs right away. For example, have a sandwich or a glass of juice. If you are dealing with type 1 diabetes, you can take in more insulin and then contact a medical professional if you don't notice that you feel better right away to solve the problem.

Ketosis is a perfectly natural process. It is one that allows you to burn through more of the fats that you burn and the ones stored in your body, rather than relying on carbs as an energy source. This is a process that has happened many times throughout your life, you just didn't realize it. But with the ketogenic diet, you are taking advantage of this process to help improve your health and lose weight.

Chapter 3: What Foods Can I Choose on the Ketogenic Diet?

When you first hear about the ketogenic diet, you will probably see that there are a ton of foods that you are supposed to avoid in order to see the best results with your health. Most people get worried when it comes to the foods they can eat and the ones they need to avoid on this diet plan because it seems extensively to give up some of their favorite foods. The good news is that the ketogenic diet encourages lots of healthy and wholesome foods, so you will still be able to eat some of your favorites, you just need to make some modifications.

One of the first questions that people have when they want to get started on the ketogenic diet is what kinds of foods they are allowed to consume, and which ones they should avoid. Some examples of foods that are acceptable on the ketogenic diet (and you should avoid all the other types of foods) include:

Seafood

Shellfish and fish are considered very friendly when you are on the ketogenic diet. Salmon and many other types of fish are going to be rich in B vitamins, selenium, and potassium, and you will notice that they are extremely low in carbs, which makes them perfect for this diet plan.

However, you will need to be careful about the shellfish in some instances. For example, most crabs and shrimp won't have any carbs, but there are other types of shellfish that are going to contain a lot of carbs in them. While you can include the other types of shellfish on the diet, you just need to be careful about how much you consume because they do contain carbs, and you don't want to eat so many that it kicks you out of the ketosis you are aiming for.

Some examples of the carb counts that come with a 3.5 ounce serving of some of the different shellfish that you need to watch out for include:

1. Clams: 5 grams
2. Mussels: 7 grams
3. Octopus: 4 grams
4. Oysters: 4 grams
5. Squid: 3 grams

You will find that there are lots of fatty fish, such as mackerel, sardines, and salmon, are going to be approved on the ketogenic diet, and they bring in the added benefit of being really high in healthy omega-3 fatty acids. Eating plenty of omega-3 fatty acids has been shown to help the brain stay sharp, can lower insulin levels, and can even increase the insulin sensitivity that is found in overweight and obese people. This nutrient can also help to reduce your risk of developing heart disease.

Because of all the great benefits of seafood, it is recommended that you consume a few servings of this in your diet each week.

Low Carb Vegetables

You will find that the majority of the carbs you consume on this diet plan are going to come from low carb vegetables. Many non-starch vegetables are going to be low in calories and carbs, while also containing a lot of the nutrients that your body needs to do well. They also contain fiber, which your body doesn't digest and absorb like other carbs. This is why you should look more at the net carb count in order to figure out what the total carbs of the item are, without the fiber.

Make sure that you know the difference between starchy and non-starchy vegetables. The non-starchy vegetables are going to have few net carbs, and you can eat plenty of these on the ketogenic diet. However, just one serving of the vegetables that are considered starchy, such as beets, yams, and potatoes, could kick you over your carb limit for the day.

You can enjoy a few servings of the non-starchy vegetables in your day. These provide you with a lot of the antioxidants and nutrients that the body needs to get throughout the day. Adding in a few with your meals, and enjoying them as a snack can help you get a lot of the nutrition that you are going to need while on the ketogenic diet.

Dairy Products

You are also able to consume some healthy sources of dairy while you are on this plan. But make sure that you are going with the higher fat versions. And you also need to make sure that you avoid the added sugars that come with these. This means that you should be careful with any product that has sugars added to it or flavoring to it. For example, if you want to eat a yogurt, don't go through and purchase the kinds that already have the fruit added in because these are going to be high in sugars. Instead, choose to go with Greek yogurt or regular yogurt and add in some of your own berries to avoid the sugar.

There are many different types of dairy products that you can choose to go with as well. You can choose to go with options like milk, cheese, sour cream, and yogurt. Just make sure that you go with the version that is full fat, and don't go with any kind that has any kind of added sugars to it.

Meat and Poultry

Next on the list is the meat and poultry. These are staples that come on the ketogenic diet. Fresh poultry and meat don't have any carbs and they are rich in the B vitamins along with some other minerals like zinc, selenium, and potassium. They also have some high-quality protein in them, which can be a great thing when you are trying to preserve your muscle mass on a low carb diet like this one.

In one study done on older women, it was found that consuming a diet that was higher in fatty meats led to those individuals having HDL cholesterol levels that were 8 percent higher compared to those on a traditional American diet, or another diet that was high carb and ow fat.

When you are picking out the types of meats and poultry that you can enjoy on the ketogenic diet, try to go with grass fed meats as much as possible. This is because the animals that are given grass will produce meat that have higher amounts of omega-3 fatty acids, and more antioxidants, compared to the animals who are fed grains and other products.

Eggs

Eggs are a very versatile and healthy food that you can enjoy on this diet plan. In addition to all of the nutrients that you can get, such as the antioxidants of zeaxanthin and lutein that can protect the health of the eyes, eggs are known to trigger hormones that can increase your feelings of fullness. They also help you to keep your levels of blood sugars stable, leading to lower amounts of calories consumed for a 24 hour period.

Even though the egg, especially the yolks, are higher in cholesterol, this doesn't mean that they are going to raise your blood cholesterol levels. In fact, it seems that eggs are able to modify the shape of LDL in a way that can actually reduce the risk that you face of heart disease, making them the perfect choice to add into your ketogenic diet plan.

Coconut and Olive Oil

To start with, we can look at coconut oil. Coconut oil has a lot of unique properties that makes it great for this kind of diet plan. To start with, it contains MCTs, or medium chain triglycerides. Unlike some of the long chain fats, these MCTs are going to be taken in by the liver and this is where they can be converted to ketones to use in the body as energy. In fat, this kind of oil has been used in order to increase the ketone levels in those who are dealing with several different nervous system and brain disorders, such as Alzheimer's.

The main fatty acid that is found in coconut oil, lauric acid, is going to be a slightly longer chain fat. It is suggested that the mixture of lauric acid and MCTs in the oil may be able to help sustain a level of ketosis in the body.

In addition, coconut oil may be able to help adults who are obese lose more weight and belly fat over all. In one study, men who consumed two tablespoons of coconut oil were able to lose one inch, on average, from their waistlines without making any other changes in their diet.

Olive oil can also provide some impressive benefits to your heart. It is high in oleic acid, a monounsaturated fat that is able to decrease several risk factors that you may experience for heart disease. In addition, extra-virgin olive oil is very high in some different antioxidants that are known as phenols. These compounds are able to go even further for protecting the health of your heart by improving how well the arteries are able to function and decreasing inflammation.

And since both of these are pure sources of fats, they can help you reach your daily requirements for fats while also not containing any carbs. It is a great base when it comes to salad dressings and other options

Nuts and Seeds

Generally, seeds and nuts are going to be healthy foods that are low in carbs and higher in fats. Eating nuts on a regular basis, especially as a nice snack, can be linked to a lower risk of depression, certain types of cancers, and heart disease, along with a few other chronic health problems. In addition, you will find that most seeds and nuts are going to be higher in fiber, which can make it easier for you to feel full with fewer calories.

Of course, most nuts are going to include some carbs in them, so you should be careful with how much and what types you want to consume. If you take on too many, it can result in too many carbs. A handful a day is usually enough to provide you with the health benefits that this provides, without having to worry about the extra carbs that are found inside.

Berries

For the most part, most of the fruits that are out there are going to be too high in carbs for you to include in the ketogenic diet. You can include them on occasion, but your consumption should be very rare, and only like one serving a day. However, berries are an exception to this rule. Berries are a great option because they are high in fiber and still low in carbs. In fact, both blackberries and raspberries are going to contain as much fiber as digestible carbs.

These tiny fruits are going to also be full of lots of antioxidants. These are the nutrients that are credited with protecting against a wide variety of diseases and reducing inflammation. You can enjoy all of the berries including strawberries, raspberries, blueberries, and blackberries on this diet plan.

Butter and Cream

Both cream and butter are soon as good fats that you can include on the ketogenic diet. They have tons of the good fats, without just trace amounts of the carbs in each serving. This is against what many traditional diet plans taught because it was believed for years that cream and butter would contribute to heart disease because they had higher levels of fat content inside. However, there have now been a few studies that show that, for most individuals, this saturated fat isn't linked to diseases of the heart.

In fact, there are studies out there that show how a moderate amount of dairy that is high in fat each day may actually be able to reduce the risk of stroke and heart attack in many individuals. Like some of the other fatty dairy products that you may enjoy on this diet plan, both cream and butter are going to be high in a substance known as conjugated linoleic acid. This is a fatty acid that you want to pay attention to because it may be able to promote fat loss.

Shirataki Noodles

These are a great substitute to noodles that can still work well with the ketogenic diet, and will ensure that you can still make some of your favorite meals on this plan. They are going to have about five calories in each serving and just one gram of carb because they are filled up with mostly water. In fact, they are a type of viscous fiber that is known as glucomannan, which is able to take in up to 50 times its own weight with water.

Viscous fiber is going to form into a gel that will slow down how quickly the food is able to move through your digestive tract. This is a great thing for those who are trying to lose weight, and it can help to decrease hunger as well as blood sugar spikes. This makes it beneficial for diabetes management and weight loss too. You can find these noodles in a variety of shapes, including linguine, fettuccini, and rice.

Unsweetened Tea and Coffee

While the majority of your liquids need to come from water to help you stay hydrated, you can enjoy tea and coffee, as long as they are unsweetened. They are healthy and free of carbs, which makes them perfect for the ketogenic diet. They do contain some caffeine in them, which will help to increase your metabolism and may be able to improve your mood, alertness and physical performance.

There have been a few studies done on these beverages, and it has been shown how tea and coffee drinkers will have a significantly reduced risk of diabetes. In fact, those with the highest tea and coffee intakes are the ones who have the lowest risk when it comes to developing diabetes.

While on the ketogenic diet, you are allowed to add in some heavy cream to the tea and coffee. But make sure that you are not adding in sugar, and that you stay away from light teas and coffees because they use the non-fat milks and the flavorings that are high in carbs.

Dark Chocolate

And finally, when you are on the ketogenic diet, you can have a little bit of cocoa powder and dark chocolate. These are both delicious sources of your antioxidants, and cocoa has even been known as a super fruit because it can provide a similar amount of antioxidants as you will get from eating other fruits, even acai berries and blueberries. And the flavanols that are found in dark chocolates could reduce your risk of heart disease simply by lowering your blood pressure and helping to make sure that the arteries are as healthy as possible.

It may be surprising that you can add dark chocolate to the ketogenic diet, but because of the benefits above, it is encouraged on occasion. However, there are a few things to keep in mind with this. First off, only pick out dark chocolate that has at least 70 percent cocoa solids. More is better in this case. And always remember that the chocolate is going to contain up to 10 grams of net carbs, so only enjoy on a special occasion.

Foods to Avoid

Now that we know a bit more about some of the tasty foods that you are allowed to consume on the ketogenic diet, it is important to take a look at some of the foods that are not allowed. Eating these kinds of foods can kick you out of ketosis and will make it hard for you to see the results that you would like on this diet plan. Some of the foods that you should avoid when you go on the ketogenic diet includes:

- Foods with sugars: sugar works the same way in the body as carbs do so eating a lot of those is bad on the ketogenic diet. You need to avoid options like soda, smoothies, cake, fruit juices, ice cream, baked goods, and candy to stay healthy.

- Starches and grains: these have a huge amount of carbs inside of them and can easily send you out of the ketosis state. Choose to avoid options like rice, cereals, and pasta and any other wheat product.

- Fruit: for the most part, you will need to limit the amount of fruit you eat on this diet because it is high in carbs and sugars. If you do enjoy some fruit on occasion, stick with options that are lower in carbs, such as berries.

- Unhealthy fats: while you do need to eat lots of fats inside this diet plan, you need to be careful that you are eating the right kinds of fats. Avoid processed fats, saturated fats, and so on to stay healthy.

- Most condiments: most condiments are bad for the ketogenic diet. These often hide their carbs and sugars and they can kick you out of the ketosis state in no time.

- Low fat products: diet products that claim they are low fat are bad for this diet. First, you need to take in more fat to make this diet work, so going low fat is not good. Second, most of these diet products are high in carbs and sugars from all the processing so it is best to avoid them to start with.

- Root vegetables: while some vegetables are fine to eat because they are low in carbs, you need to watch out for the root vegetables. These include options like potatoes, carrots, sweet potatoes, and parsnips.

- Legumes and beans: these are high in carbs and while other diets praise how great they are for keeping you full, they are a big part of the problem you are trying to solve with the ketogenic diet. Some legumes and beans that you must avoid on this diet include peas, lentils, kidney beans, and chickpeas.

When it comes to following the ketogenic diet, you will want to make sure that you are picking out foods that are very low in carbs. This means that you are going to need to cut down on some of the foods that you might have enjoyed more in the past. Limiting your consumption of breads, pastas, and many types of fruits, along with the baked goods, can go a long way in helping you to lose weight and feel amazing.

The ketogenic diet may seem a bit more restrictive than what you may be used to on your traditional meal plan, but the results are very powerful. When you are ready to get started on this meal plan, make sure that you are writing out a good grocery list and sticking with it to see the best results.

Chapter 4: The Amazing Health Benefits of the Ketogenic Diet

The next topic that we need to look at is all the great health benefits that you can enjoy when it comes to the ketogenic diet. In addition to the great weight loss that you can enjoy when you get started with this diet plan, there are a bunch of other health benefits that can make it worth your time. While there are some people who are against a ketogenic diet and feel that it is a bad choice for your health, looking through the studies and the research that have been done on this topic can help show that it is actually a very healthy plan to get started on. Let's take a look at some of the health benefits that come with the ketogenic diet and why you should consider adding it into your own life as well.

Can Reduce Your Appetite

One of the hardest things about getting started with any kind of diet plan is the hunger. You start out with all of the best intentions, and then find that the hunger will limit you and make it almost impossible to stick with your plan. Hunger is very much the worst side effect of dieting. It is often one of the main reasons why people will feel miserable and then give up.

However, when you switch over from your high carb diet to one that is lower in carbs, this is going to lead to an automatic reduction in your appetite overall. Studies consistently show that when you cut out how many carbs you are consuming and learn how to eat more protein and fat, you will actually end up eating far fewer calories. This can make it even easier to lose the weight that you want.

Lose More Fat in the Belly

While you are able to lose weight with the ketogenic diet, you will find that what is even better is that you are able to lose more fat around the stomach as well. Not all of the fat that is stored throughout the body is going to be the same. Often the location where this fat is placed is going to affect how much it changes your health and your own personal risk for disease.

There are two types of fat on the body. The first one is the subcutaneous fat, or the fat that is found under the skin. And then there is the visceral fat, which is the kind that is found in the abdominal cavity. Visceral fat is often going to lodge itself around your organs and having an excess amount of this can be associated with resistance to insulin and inflammation throughout the body. It may even be the main cause of metabolic dysfunction that is found throughout the Western world today.

The neat thing about the ketogenic diet, and other low carb diets, is that they are effective at reducing the amount of this fat in the body. In fact, a larger amount of fat that people lose on these low carb diets seems to come from the abdominal cavity. And if you are able to lose enough of this fat in your stomach and around the organs, it can help reduce your risk of type 2 diabetes and heart disease.

A Drop in Your Triglycerides

When you go on the ketogenic diet, you will notice that there is a drop in the number of triglycerides in the body. These are basically fat molecules that like to circulate all around the bloodstream. It is known that having a high fasting amount of these fat molecules, or higher levels in the blood after not eating all night, can be a strong risk factor for heart disease.

There are two main drivers that are going to cause you to have a higher level of triglycerides in the body. This includes being sedentary and eating too many carbs. This is especially potent if you eat too much of the simple sugar fructose. When you are able to cut out the number of carbs you are consuming, you will also be able to see a big reduction in your blood triglycerides as well.

Can Reduce Your Insulin Levels and Your Blood Sugar Levels

Following a low carb diet, like the ketogenic diet, can be helpful for those individuals who are dealing with resistance to insulin and diabetes. And since millions of people throughout the world are dealing with these conditions, this is definitely something that should be explored even more.

Studies that have been done so far show that cutting out the number of carbs that you consume can really help to lower both your insulin levels and your blood sugar levels by quite a bit. Depending on the severity of these two conditions, and how well the individual is able to stick with the diet, you may be able to reduce the amount of insulin you take in. For example, some of those who were suffering from diabetes who started on the ketogenic diet, or another low carb diet, were able to reduce how much insulin they had to take each day by almost 50 percent right away.

In another study that took a look at diabetes and the ketogenic diet done on those who had type 2 diabetes, it was found that 95 percent of these individuals were able to either reduce, or completely eliminate, the medication they took to lower glucose medication within a six month period.

These studies may change the way that we handle diabetes in the future. Right now, it seems that those who are dealing with these conditions could see some vast improvements if they were just able to follow the diet for a little bit. However, if you are taking any kind of medication for your blood sugar, make sure to talk with your doctor before you make any changes in how many carbs you consume. It is possible that your dosage will need to be adjusted and changed in order to prevent issues with hypoglycemia.

Can Help to Lower Your Blood Pressure

For those who are dealing with higher blood pressure, it is important to get those numbers down. Allowing your blood pressure to stay high, and not taking the right steps to fix this issue, can result in a number of health problems overall, including heart disease and stroke. It can even result in kidney failure if the levels get high enough and don't get taken care of.

There are a number of steps that you can take to help lower your blood pressure. But one of the most effective methods that you can work with is to go on a low carb diet like the ketogenic diet. If you can follow this diet for just a bit, you will find that it is a great way to lower your blood pressure levels and this can help you to reduce the risk of these diseases, prolonging your life.

Fights off Metabolic Syndrome

Another condition that many people in American and around the world may deal with is metabolic syndrome. This is a type of condition that can be associated with the amount of risk that you have for heart disease and diabetes. It is not really just one disease though. Instead, it is more of a collection of symptoms that all come together, and all of them can be bad for your overall health. Some of the symptoms that can come from dealing with metabolic syndrome may include:

Lower levels of the good cholesterol through the body
A high number of triglycerides, especially the fasting levels.
Elevated blood pressure that is hard to bring down through exercise and other means.
Obesity around the stomach.
An elevated number of fasting blood sugar levels.

All of these can cause some damage to your heart if you are not careful about it. Implementing a low carb diet like the ketogenic diet can help to deal with all of these symptoms in an effective way, and can make metabolic syndrome a thing of the past for those who are dealing with it. In fact, under the ketogenic diet, it is possible that you can greatly reduce, or at least eliminate, these conditions.

Helps with Your Levels of Cholesterol

There are many ways that the ketogenic diet is able to help with your cholesterol levels. Like we talked about before, it is able to help improve your levels of triglycerides throughout the body. This can work to help out your cholesterol levels as well. But there are a few other parts of the equation that come into play as well.

The ketogenic diet not only works to help improve your triglyceride levels, it can also help you to reduce the number of bad cholesterol while also increasing the amount of good cholesterol. When all of these factors come together, you are able to help improve the body and see some amazing results.

It Can Do Some Wonders for Several Brain Disorders

Many people decide to go on the ketogenic diet because it is able to help improve the brain in many different manners. To start, when you go on the ketogenic diet, you are going to see a big improvement in how clear your mind is. You will be able to think more clearly, be more creative, and not have to worry so much about the brain fog and other issues that may bother you.

But the ketogenic diet can take it even further than that. In fact, it can help out with many serious mental conditions including Parkinson's disease, Alzheimer's disease, and even childhood epilepsy.

Your brain needs to have glucose to help it survive. There are just some parts of the brain that only know how to burn up this kind of sugar. But the good news is that when you are on this low carb diet, the liver is able to produce glucose out of the protein that you consume, so you won't have to worry about starving out that part of the brain when you stop eating so many carbs.

With that said, there is a big part of the brain that is also able to burn up ketones. These ketones, if you remember, are formed during starvation, such as going on a fast, or when the intake of carbs into the body is low, such as when you go on the ketogenic diet. This is a mechanism that helps to run the ketogenic diet, and it has been used for many years in order to treat epilepsy in children who aren't responding well to other drug treatments.

In many cases, going on the ketogenic diet, or another one that is very similar, was able to cure children of epilepsy. In fact, in one study, more than half of the children who went on this diet were able to see more than a 50 percent reduction in the number of seizures that they experienced. What is even better is that about 16 percent of the participants in the study were able to become seizure free at the end.

This is great news for those who are suffering from seizures and who haven't been able to respond to some of the other treatment methods out there. It can reduce their symptoms and makes a big difference in their quality of life as well. Because of the great results that have been shown in this study and more, many studies are now trying to take a look into some of the other effects that the ketogenic diet can have on the brain and whether or not it is able to help with some other common diseases such as Parkinson's and Alzheimer's.

The Diet Can Help You Lose Weight

One of the number one reasons that people choose to go on the ketogenic diet is because it can help them to lose weight. There are a number of reasons for this. First, you will start to take in fewer calories overall when you are on this diet plan. Foods that are low in carbs and high in fats and good proteins are going to be more filling, while holding fewer calories. Many of those who decide to go on the ketogenic diet will notice some big improvements in how hungry they are, and this helps them to reduce the number of calories they eat overall.

This kind of diet plan is also able to speed up the metabolism as well. Those who go on this diet plan are replacing glucose, in the form of sugars and carbs, as their main source of energy. This can do some wonders for helping you to speed up the metabolism, eat fewer calories, and still feel like you are taking in enough to eat.

Another benefit that can help you to lose weight is that the ketogenic diet is going to help increase your energy levels. The body can actually thrive on healthy fats, and you may find that without the afternoon crash that comes from carbs and sugars, you have more energy in your day and can get more done. When you put that energy to good use and learn how to be more active and exercise more throughout the day, it is going to lead to some more results with losing weight on the ketogenic diet.

As you can see, there are a lot of great benefits that come with following the ketogenic diet. Because you are reducing the amount of unhealthy and bad foods that you consume and you replace them with lots of healthy and wholesome foods, it can do a lot of wonders for your overall health. When you are tired of being sick and tired, make sure to check out the ketogenic diet and see just how much it can do to improve your health and how you feel.

Chapter 5: Are There Any Precautions I Should Take with the Ketogenic Diet?

Before you decide to go on the keto diet it is important to realize that even though there are some positives that come with this diet plan, there are also a few negatives that you should know about as well. The ketogenic diet is generally seen as a safe option for those who want to lose weight and improve their health, but during the first few weeks on this kind of diet plan, you may notice that there are a few side effects that you need to be careful about. The good news is that for the most part, these side effects will fade after the first week or so, so getting through them isn't too difficult. Let's take a look at some of the negative side

The Keto Flu

Another issue that can come up when you are dealing with the ketogenic diet is something known as the keto flu. This is something that can show up in the first week or so of being on this eating plan. Since you are putting some different foods in your body, and removing some of your old favorites that your body had relied on in the past, you will find that the body needs a bit of time to adjust to this new eating plan.

The body is used to having carbs as a form of energy. This is what you have been feeding it for years, and when you take away the majority of the carbs that you consume, you will find that the body gets worn out and tired. When you follow a very low carb diet, the body is going to work on burning through ketones, the byproducts that come from breaking down the fats, instead of carbs.

When this process happens, the body needs some time to adjust to the new method, and in the process you may have some symptoms that seem similar to the flue. This is because the switch is going to catch the body off guard, and it may feel sick until it is able to regulate itself and adapt to the new process. Some of the symptoms that you may experience when you are dealing with the keto flu includes weakness, headaches, muscles cramps, constipation, vomiting, and nausea.

The severity of the keto flu is going to depend on how much you relied on the carbs ahead of this diet plan and how long it takes you to get into ketosis. This can be hard when you just want to deal with some of the cravings that come with this diet plan. But if you make sure that you sit back and relax and take it easy during the time you are experiencing the keto flu, you will be able to see some relief.

Sugar Cravings

You will find that in the first few weeks of being on the ketogenic diet, you are going to experience quite a few sugar cravings along he way. Many people find that these cravings can make it really hard to stick with the diet plan and since they are for high sugar foods, rather than for the high fat foods that you should be eating on this diet plan, they can sometimes pose a big challenge to your personal willpower.

The brain is sending out these cravings because it wants to have the easy source of fuel that comes from carbs. And since you are not able to get the fat converted to energy right away, you may find that it is hard to avoid those cravings and you may feel an intense desire for the sugar and high carb foods in the beginning.

To avoid this issue, take some time to eat high fat foods, relax, and try to use as little energy as possible during this time. Remember that if you are able to make it through the first few weeks of this diet plan, you will be able to get relief from the bad cravings and the ketogenic diet will be much easier to stick with.

Drowsiness and Dizziness

During the first week or so on this diet plan, you will often feel drowsy and dizzy because you are going to be low on energy. Some people experience an extra amount of dizziness when they stand up because of blood pressure dysregulation and inappropriate cortisol response. You can take it easy and sleep a bit extra in the beginning, and take some extra time to stand up as your body adjusts.

A Reduction in Your Strength and Physical Performance

If you were used to doing an intense workout before you started this diet plan, you may want to take it easy in the beginning. You are going to be short on some of the energy that you are used to enjoying. You may feel a bit weak and tired in the beginning as well. During this time, the body is adapting and learning how to utilize a new fuel source, one that it hasn't used in the past. The muscles including the brain, contain a lot of mitochondria for producing energy, and now it needs to learn how it is supposed to work with ketones as an energy source.

During this time, you may feel that there is a significant drop in the amount of strength that you have, and your ability to exert physical energy is going to be reduced as one of the short term side effects of this diet plan. The good news is that once you are adapted to this plan, you will be able to see big improvements, and your physical performance and strength will increase even more than what you saw before this diet plan.

Low Libido

Since you are going to kick out a lot of the carbs that you usually eat when you go on this diet plan, your body may be dealing with less energy than before. And ultimately, this can lead to a lower sex drive. In addition to lower amounts of energy, switching from the traditional diet to one that is low carb and high fat could cause some imbalances in your hormones.

It has been shown how too few carbs in your diet can cause some troubles with your thyroid. The thyroid is responsible for regulating all the hormones throughout the body. Because of this, you may find that you are just not in the mood for sex. Plus, when you are first getting started with this diet plan, you won't feel the best (remember the keto flu), so you will feel even less like you want to do any activity that will require a lot of energy from you.

While the ketogenic diet can be a great plan to go on, there are a few side effects that you will want to be careful. You want to make sure that you are aware of these side effects, and then learn how to handle them and take it easy, in order to get the full benefits that come with this diet plan.

How to Avoid Hypoglycemia

With most of the side effects that we talked about before, the main cause of this is hypoglycemia. If you are able to deal with this issue, you will be able to improve your health and you can make the start of this diet plan easier on everyone. Some of the strategies that you can use in order to deal with the issues of hypoglycemia and the side effects that you have include:

1. Eat at least every four hours. In the beginning of the ketogenic diet, make sure that you are eating every three to four hours. This can ensure that you are fully satiated and that your blood sugars stay balanced.

2. Drink beverages that are full of minerals: Instead of just drinking plain water, for example, you can add in some mineral rich beverages between your meals. This could be a keto approved electrolyte drink or some organic broths.

3. Foods that are full of minerals and are hydrating: Consume plenty of meals that have a lot of minerals and are hydrating. This can help ensure that you don't become dehydrated, which can make the experience on this diet plan difficult.

4. Use some exogenous ketones: Exogenous ketones are a good way to train the body to use ketones for fuel before the body gets used to making its own. They are able to also help out with the hypoglycemic responses by providing you with ketones that can then be used as energy.

5. Supplement with some magnesium: If you follow some of the strategies above and you still feel some of the symptoms that we listed above, you may want to add a magnesium supplement into your regimen. You can take some magnesium a few times a day to help you get through this process.

The good news about these side effects is that they are usually going to be temporary and you don't have to worry about them lasting for a long time. If you can make it through the adapting phase and make it through a few weeks on this diet plan, you will see some improvements to your health and the majority, if not all, of these side effects will fade.

Chapter 6: The Great Benefits of the Slow Cooker

There are many different utensils and appliances that you are able to use in your kitchen. Some of them are more traditional and may include the oven. Some may work with an instant pot in order to provide you a pressure cooked meal in just a few minutes. There is also the microwave, the air fryer and so much more. But one of the best options that you can choose to use to get dinner on the table and still maintain the nutrition and the flavor includes:

A slow cooker can be really helpful when you want to get a delicious meal in at the beginning of the day and then have it waiting for you and your family at the end of the day. There are a ton of different benefits that come with using the slow cooker and these include:

- Having a meal already at home, waiting for you in the slow cooker, can eliminate any of the temptations that you may have to order take out. This can help you get more nutrition, saves you money, and can help you stay on the ketogenic diet.

- Slow cookers are usually going to allow for one step preparation. This means that you can just grab the ingredients and throw them all in with little preparation. This saves you time and can cut down on the amount of clean up that you need to do.

- You can use your slow cooker throughout the whole year. Many people love having them in the winter to make some welcoming soups. And they also work well in the summer because you can cook a good meal without having to overheat the kitchen with the oven.

- As a result of the long and low-temperature cooking, the slow cooker is great for tenderizing some of the less-expensive cuts of meat compared to other forms of cooking.

- A slow cooker can bring out all of the flavor that is found in foods. A wide variety of foods can be coked in the slow cooker, including casseroles, stews, soups, and one pot meals.

- A slow cooker is going to use a lot less electricity compared to an over.

As you can see, there are a lot of benefits that come with the slow cooker. You can save money, avoid going out to eat as often, lose weight, and so much more. And since it can be used during any time of the year that you would like, there is never a reason why you wouldn't want to pull out the slow cooker and make some of your favorite recipes today.

Knowing Your Slow Cooker

Most slow cookers are going to come with either two or three settings. When you are using the low setting, you will usually rely on cooking for between six to ten hours. The high setting can usually get the food done within four to six hours. If you can, it is usually best to use the high setting for the first hour of the cooking time and then switch over to the low setting to finish up. But, if you have to leave the home, sticking with the lower setting is just fine.

Slow cookers are going to vary in size based on what you need and you can usually find them between one to seven quarts. Smaller slow cookers are good for dips or sauces if you need, and then the larger cookers are going to be good for some larger cuts of meats or some soups. If you are trying to cook for four or fewer people, a 3.5 to 4 quart size slow cooker is the best option, and the five to seven, or even bigger, slow cookers are best if you plan to cook for more people or you want some leftovers.

No matter what you would like to cook, or how many people you would like to cook for, the slow cooker is able to work for everyone. It can make cooking easier, especially when you are trying to work with the ketogenic diet.

Tips and Safety for the Slow Cooker

If you haven't had much time to use the slow cooker, and you are a bit worried about leaving an appliance on all day when you aren't even home, you do have a few options. You could use alternate hours, such as when you are sleeping for example, or cool down foods when they are finished. Some of the other tips and safety rules that you are able to use when it comes to a slow cooker includes:

- For cleanup that is easy, and to take good care of your slow cooker, make sure to rub the inside of it with some oil or some cooking spray ahead of time. You can also consider going with some liners for the slow cooker to make cleanup a bit easier as well.

- If you can, try to thaw out frozen poultry and meat before you move it over to cook in the slow cooker. To ensure that the cooking process is complete, do not add frozen meat into the slow cooker if you can help it.

- Fill up the slow cooker so that it is more than half full, and no more than two-thirds full. Cooking either too little or too much food in the slow cooker is going to change the cooking time, the quality of the meal, and even the safety.

- Because vegetables are going to cook at a slower rate in the slow cooker compared to poultry and meat, make sure that the vegetables are placed inside first. Then you can add the meat on top of the vegetables. Top it all with the liquid that you are going to use, such as the sauce, the broth, or the water.

- Make sure that you add in the liquid, such as the sauce, the water, or the broth, that the recipe suggests. Because liquids are not going to boil in the slow cooker, due to its low heat, you can reduce liquids by one third to one half when you are taking a non-slow cooker recipe over to a slow cooker one.

- If possible, you should try to set the slow cooker on a high setting for the first hour. Then, when the time is up, you can move it to the right setting, or down to the low setting if the recipe calls for it.

- Make sure that the lid stays in place when you are cooking. If the lid is not secure, or if you remove the lid at all during this time, it is going to slow down your cooking time. Every time that you lift up the lid, it can take off up to 20 minutes of the cooking time.

- Add in any grains that you want to cook, such as the pasta, at the end of the cooking process. Adding them at the beginning is going to result in them becoming mushy. You can even cook the pasta, or some other grains like rice, on their own, and then add them in right before you serve the rest of the dish.

- Add in the cream, cheese, and milk during the last hour to make sure that you don't end up with curdling.

- When it comes to some of the softer vegetables, like zucchini, mushrooms, and tomatoes, make sure that these are added during the last 30 to 45 minutes of the cooking process. Adding them in too early can end up with them being too soft and it can ruin the recipe.

Using your slow cooker is meant to be easy. When many families are busy and need to get a quick meal on the table, or they know they won't have time that night to make a home cooked meal and spend all that time in the kitchen, they will often turn to the slow cooker in order to get things done. In many cases, the recipes that you find with the slow cooker are going to be one step, which means you can just grab the ingredients that the recipe calls for and then throw them all in, place the lid on top, and have it all cook for you. What could be easier when it comes to starting the ketogenic diet and seeing some amazing results quickly.

Chapter 7: Tips for Following the Ketogenic Diet While Using the Slow Cooker

The ketogenic diet is one of the best options for you to go with when you are ready to lose weight and improve your health. However, it can be a difficult diet plan to go with. You have to give up all of your favorite carb loaded foods in the hopes of seeing some benefits with how healthy you can feel. However, there are a few things that you can do to help make the ketogenic diet easier, and to ensure you will see the results that you want. These tips include:

Do it with Friends

Doing the diet plan with your friends along to help can make a big difference in whether you are going to see the results that you want or not. Find someone who has the same goals as you do, or someone who is on the ketogenic diet as well, who can go on the journey with you, encourage you along, and help you to really see results.

The friend you are working with does not have to be on the ketogenic diet if you can't find someone with that same goal as you. Someone who is working towards weight loss, even if it is with another diet plan, or someone who has another goal they are trying to reach can be a great asset to helping you as well.

This is the person that you are going to turn to when things get tough and you need that extra bit of encouragement to get through the day. This is that person you can go to the gym with, share recipes with, and explain the tips that are working the best for each of you. You will be amazed at how much easier it is to stay focused and dedicated to the weight loss program, to any program, when you have someone by your side to encourage along the journey.

You do need to remember to be that person of encouragement to your partner as well. It isn't fair for them to give out all the encouragement while you sit by and hope it all works out well. When they have a bad day, be there for them. When they want to skip a day at the gym, make sure to get them out of the house and help them get the best workout in ever.

You both need to be there for each other through this adventure because it is hard. But when you work together and hold each other accountable, it is much easier to see the results that you want.

Slowly Eliminate Some of the Carbs That You are Consuming

For some people, it can be hard to give up all of those carbs all of a sudden. When you are eating up to 200 or more grams of carbs each day, and then you need to eliminate down to 50 grams a day or more, it can be a shock to the body. And some people just won't be able to do it very well. If you try this for a few days and it just doesn't seem to be working for you, consider adding more in for the beginning, and then change it down later on.

For example, if you monitor your carbs and you see that you take in 200 grams a day, you may want to try out a week where you eliminate to 150 grams a day. Then do a week with 100 grams a day. And then reduce down to 50 grams. And if you need to go down even further than this, that fourth week will be a good option for you to choose.

Going slowly like this can make a big difference. It allows you to take it a bit slower. You can adjust to eating fewer carbs in a slower fashion, a more gentle fashion, compared to some of the other methods of jumping in, and you may not have to deal with as many of the negative side effects as before.

Plan Ahead a Little

The slow cooker can be your best friend when you are getting started with a new diet plan. It allows you to put meals in during the morning, and then when you get home, there is a nice home cooked meal for you to enjoy. But in order to make this happen, you need to actually plan ahead. The slow cooker and the ease that it brings to your life isn't going to do much if you wait until you get home to even think about what you want for dinner.

When you get up in the morning, think about how busy that day may be, and whether or not you would like to use a slow cooker meal to make things easier. You can then set things out to ensure that you are able to get all of the food on the table and ready to go. You can then gather all of the ingredients and get it thrown in at the right time to have supper on the table on time.

Set Goals

How are you going to know that you are getting somewhere if you don't have some goals to help you out? Before you get started on this diet plan, think of the goals that you would like to succeed and then divide them up into little goals that you can accomplish along the way. This is one of the best ways to stay motivated and ensure that you are going to see the results that you want.

Make sure that when you are setting goals, you go with ones that are manageable for you. Just because someone else has the time and energy to do two hour workouts a day doesn't mean this should be your goal. Maybe you can choose to lose so much weight by a certain time, or cut down your carb intake so much a week. Think about what you want to get out of the ketogenic diet the most, and then make this part of your plans.

Looking at Labels

While this list is a good place for you to get started when you are using the ketogenic diet, you still need to be proactive about what you are eating with this diet plan. You should take some time to look at the nutritional label when you want to purchase something and want to see if you are able to eat it. The lists above are guidelines to help you, but they don't go through all of the foods that you will find on your next trip to the store.

After some time, you will find that you will recognize the items in your store that fit into the ketogenic diet. But for the first bit, you will need to learn how to read through the labels and determine if the carb content is low enough and the fat content is high enough. You can take a cheat sheet around that has all the ingredients that you are looking for and how they should separate out to make this easier. You will soon learn which brands of each product fit on the ketogenic diet and it will make things a bit easier down the road, but in the beginning, you will find that your trips to the grocery store may last a bit longer than you are used to.

It may seem like a pain to have to go through all the labels when you first get started, but how are you going to determine the best foods to go with otherwise? You might know that you can have cream, but each type of cream is going to have different ingredients inside and without looking at the label, you could easily take in more of the carbs in a healthy looking product than what is allowed on this diet plan. Always take the time to look at what is on the label of all the food products you are eating and see exactly what ingredients are inside to ensure you are getting everything that you need inside, and nothing that you should be avoiding.

Workout with the Diet

If you really want a chance to burn off some of the extra fat that is on your midsection, it is time to add some working out to the diet plan. The ketogenic diet is one of the best diets for losing weight, but having a good workout plan, such as doing some cardio and weight lifting most days of the week, will really make a difference in your results.

Once you have made the goals that you would like to follow, stick them in an area where you are able to see them best. Often on the fridge or the mirror in the bathroom are good choices, but find a place that is the best for you to se these each day.

Hold yourself accountable, even if that means telling other people about what you are doing so that they check in and make you work harder. These goals should motivate you towards a better you so have some fun, pick a goal that is a little bit challenging but manageable if you work hard, and then get to work!

Now, when you first get started on the ketogenic diet, you should take the first few weeks off. You may be all motivated and ready to go, but if you jump on the mal plan too quickly during this time, it can cause some issues. You will probably be tired and worn out, and you may even have some issues with the keto flu, so taking it easy and learning how your body will respond to the diet plan is very important.

Once that time period is over, you will find that it is easier to get started on a workout plan and still see results. Most people find that doing intense aerobic exercises are hard on this diet still because they need the easy source of glucose to keep you going. But you can choose to either go with a different form of working out, or you can choose to work with cyclical or another form of the ketogenic diet to ensure you are able to get the results that you want without causing any injury.

Make a Meal Plan

Another idea that you may want to try out is to develop your own meal plan. This is a great way to take into account the different types of macro nutrients that you are supposed to take in and then you won't have to worry about it during the week. Some people choose to make a meal plan for the week and others are happy with doing a whole month to save time.

The meal plan is going to work to encourage you to stay on the diet. When you are tired and hungry, you won't have to think about what you need to make, it will be ready for you right then and there. We will provide you with a 30-day meal plan for this diet to help make things a little bit easier so you can really see some results while still having time for other activities in your day.

When it comes to being on the ketogenic diet, it is important to ensure that you are on the right track right from the very beginning. The ketogenic diet can be a hard one to work with and if you aren't careful, you may fall off and lose the state of ketosis that you want to be in.

Sometimes one of the hardest parts that comes with starting the ketogenic diet is making sure that you are doing it the right way. This guidebook does come with a meal plan that you can follow in order to ensure this diet plan is easier than ever for you to start on and stick with.

Starting on the ketogenic diet is a great meal plan that can help you to improve the health of your heart, lose weight, get more energy, reduce diabetes and so much more. And when you combine it together with the slow cooker, you are going to get even better results. Make sure to follow the tips above to ensure that you are getting the most out of your ketogenic journey.

Chapter 8: Your 21 Day Meal Plan for Faster Results

Day 1:	Day 2:	Day 3:	Day 4:
Breakfast: Bacon and Spiced Egg Bake Lunch: Beef Mince and Sausage Chili Dinner: Meat Lover's Pizza	Breakfast: Almond and Ricotta Cheese Pancakes Lunch: Lemon Butter Fish Dinner: Beef Shank	Breakfast: Cheesy Omelet Lunch: Salmon and Garlic Greens Dinner: Stuffed Chicken Breasts	Breakfast: Salmon and Asparagus Lunch: Coconut Fish Curry Dinner: Beef Lasagna
Day 5	Dy 6:	Day 7	Day 8:
Breakfast: Toasted Granola Lunch: Bacon and Fish Soup Dinner: Lamb Curry	Breakfast: Ricotta Sausage Cakes Lunch: Mozzarella Shrimp Parcels Dinner: Butter Chicken	Breakfast: Stuffed Breakfast peppers Lunch: Pork Chops Dinner: Whole Chicken for Dinner	Breakfast: Berry Cheat Treats Lunch: Paprika Drumsticks Dinner: Pork Roast
Day 9:	Day 10:	Day 11:	Day 12:
Breakfast: Mushroom Melters Lunch: Beef Pot Roast Dinner: Stuffed Beef Packets	Breakfast: Hazelnut and Chocolate Pancakes Lunch: Tuna Steaks Dinner: Salmon Cake	Breakfast: Cauliflower Breakfast Cake Lunch: Spinach and Chicken Stew Dinner: Sausage and Prawn Slow Cooker Casserole	Breakfast: Keto Big Breakfast Lunch: Layered Cheeseburger Stew Dinner: Meat Lovers' Pizza

Day 13: Breakfast: Cheesy Omelet Lunch: Beef Mince and Sausage Chili Dinner: Beef Shank	Day 14: Breakfast: Berry Cheat Treats Lunch: Lemon Butter Fish Dinner: Stuffed Chicken Breasts	Day 15: Breakfast: Mushroom Melters Lunch: Pork Chops Dinner: Beef Lasagna	Day 16: Breakfast: Stuffed Breakfast peppers Lunch: Salmon and Garlic Greens Dinner: Lamb Curry
Day 17: Breakfast: Toasted Granola Lunch: Mozzarella Shrimp Parcels Dinner: Butter Chicken	Day 18: Breakfast: Ricotta Sausage Cakes Lunch: Paprika Drumsticks Dinner: Meat Lovers Pizza	Day 19: Breakfast: Salmon and Asparagus Lunch: Tuna Steaks Dinner: Whole Chicken for Dinner	Day 20: Breakfast: Almond and Ricotta Cheese Pancakes Lunch: Beef Pot Roast
Day 21 Breakfast: Keto Big Breakfast Lunch: Fish Curry Dinner: Sausage and Prawn Slow Cooker Casserole			

Chapter 9: Slow Cooker Early Morning Breakfasts

Bacon and Spiced Egg Bake

What's inside:

- Chopped parsley
- Mixed spices of cumin, chili powder, and paprika (.5 tsp.)
- Streaky bacon (4 slices)
- Eggs (4)

How to make:

1. Take out your slow cooker and drizzle in some olive oil.
2. In a small bowl, lightly beat the eggs together and then add in the spices, stirring to combine.
3. Lay the bacon slices out on the bottom of your slow cooker. Pour the egg mixture on the bacon.
4. Add the lid to the top of the slow cooker and then set the temperature to a low setting.
5. After an hour, the egg will set. Heat up a bit of oil for the frying pan and then transfer the eggs and bacon in one piece over to the skillet.
6. Cook this until the bacon can become crispy. Serve on a few plates with a bit of parsley.

Almond and Ricotta Cheese Pancakes

What's inside:

- Cinnamon (1 tsp.)
- Vanilla (1 tsp.)
- Ground almonds (.5 c.)
- Eggs (2)
- Ricotta cheese (1 c.)

How to make:

1. Take out a bowl and mix the salt, cinnamon, vanilla, ground almonds, eggs, and ricotta cheese until nice and combined.
2. Take out the slow cooker and then drizzle the coconut oil inside. Place dollops of the pancake batter into the slow cooker. It is fine if they run together just a bit.
3. Add the lid to the slow cooker and turn the temperature to a low setting.
4. After one hour, you can flip the pancakes around once. Cook for another hour before serving with some fresh berries.

Cheesy Omelet

What's inside:

- Grated cheddar (.5 c.)
- Chopped spinach (2 c.)
- Eggs (4)

How to make:

1. To start this recipe, take out the spinach and rinse it off. Place into a bowl that is microwave safe and cover before adding to the microwave. Cook for a minute until it has time to wilt.
2. At this time, squeeze out the moisture that is in the spinach and then chop it up a bit.
3. In a second bowl, beat the eggs along with the pepper, salt, cheese, and spinach.
4. Take out the slow cooker, drizzle in the oil. Pour the spinach and egg mixture into the pot. Add the lid on top and then set the temperature to a low setting.
5. After an hour, the egg should be set to your liking and you can serve this with a side of bacon and some herbs.

Salmon and Asparagus

What's inside:

- Smoked salmon (3 oz.)
- Fresh herbs (2 tsp.)
- Butter (3 Tbsp.)
- Dried chili flakes (1 tsp.)
- Crushed garlic cloves (2)
- Asparagus spears (20)

How to make:

1. For this recipe, take out the slow cooker and place some oil into the slow cooker. Add the asparagus into the bottom and sprinkle on the pepper, salt, chili, and garlic.
2. Add a bit more of the olive oil on top of the asparagus. Place the lid on top of the pot and set this to the high setting.
3. After two hours of cooking, the asparagus is done and you can place on a plate while it is hot.
4. While the asparagus is cooking, you can prepare your herb butter by combining together the pepper, salt, herbs, and butter.
5. Drape the smoked salmon on top of the asparagus and serve with the butter before enjoying.

Toasted Granola

What's inside:

- Cinnamon (1 tsp.)
- Salt (1 tsp.)
- Melted coconut oil (3 Tbsp.)
- Mixed seeds (1 c.)
- Mixed nuts (2 c.)

How to make:

1. To start this recipe, bring out a big bowl and add together the cinnamon, salt, coconut oil, seeds, and nuts together. Stir around to make sure the seeds and nuts are well coated.
2. Tip this nut and seed mixture into the slow cooker and then let the temperature be set to a high setting.
3. After two hours, the nut and see mixture should be done. You can let it cool down and store in a large jar or sprinkle over some yogurt and enjoy as a snack.

Ricotta Sausage Cakes

What's inside:

- Eggs (2)
- Sausage, sliced (2)
- Chopped baby spinach (1 c.)
- Ricotta cheese (1.5 c.)

How to make:

1. Heat up a bit of oil in a skillet. When the oil is warm, add in the sausage pieces and cook until they are browned.
2. Take out a bowl and add in the pepper, salt, eggs, sausage pieces, spinach, and ricotta cheese. Mix together well.
3. Drizzle a bit of the olive oil in the slow cooker. Shape your ricotta and sausage mixture into eight cakes and add them to the slow cooker.
4. Place the lid on top of the pot and then set it to a high setting. After one hour, turn the patties over and cook a bit longer.
5. After another hour, you can take the cakes out and serve them with some of your favorite toppings.

Stuffed Breakfast Peppers

What's inside:

- Chopped bacon (2 slices)
- Baby spinach, chopped (2 c.)
- Chunks of feta cheese (3 oz.)
- Beaten eggs (3)
- Red peppers (4)

How to make:

1. Take out a smaller bowl and mix together the pepper, salt, bacon pieces, spinach, feta cheese, and eggs.
2. Now you can prepare your peppers. You can cut around the stalk and then remove it. Reach into the peppers and get rid of the seeds inside.
3. Try to evenly pour the mixture inside of each of these prepared peppers. They may only be half full when you are done.
4. Drizzle some of the oil into the slow cooker and place your peppers into the pot, propping them up with each other to make sure they stay upright.
5. Add the lid on top of the pot and then select the High temperature. After two hours of cooking, take the peppers out of the slow cooker and serve while they are hot.

Berry Cheat Treats

What's inside:

- Melted coconut oil (1 tsp.)
- Cinnamon (.5 tsp.)
- Chopped almonds (.75 c.)
- Cream cheese (.5 lb.)
- Chopped berries (2 c.)

How to make:

1. To start this recipe, take out a bowl and combine together the cinnamon, egg, cream cheese, and berries. Take the almonds out and spread them onto a plate.
2. Roll your berry mixture into 18 even balls and then roll it into the chopped almonds to coat all the way around.
3. Take out the slow cooker and then rub some of the melted coconut oil. Place the berry balls into the bottom of the slow cooker and add the lid on top.
4. After two hours, the balls will be done. You can take them out of the oven and leave on a cooling rack before storing in the fridge until later.

Ham and Broccoli Casserole

What's inside:

- Butter (1 Tbsp.)
- Beaten eggs (10)
- Heavy cream (1 c.)
- Cheddar cheese (1.5 c.)
- Pepper
- Salt
- Parmesan cheese (.33 c.)
- Diced ham (1 c.)
- Broccoli florets (16 oz.)
- Diced yellow onion (.5)

How to make:

1. Take out a slow cooker and grease the bottom with some butter. Add in half a cup of the cheddar cheese inside along with some salt, pepper, egg, parmesan cheese, and heavy cream.
2. Whisk this all together well inside the slow cooker before stirring in the ham, broccoli, and onion. Sprinkle on the rest of the cheddar cheese.
3. Place the lid on the slow cooker and then set it to the high temperature. After three hours, the dish is done and you can serve warm.

Poblano Cheese Frittata

What's inside:

- Eggs (4)
- Half and half (1 c.)
- Green chilies (10 oz.)
- Salt (1 tsp.)
- Cumin (.5 tsp.)
- Shredded cheese (1 c.)
- Chopped cilantro (.25 c.)

How to make:

1. Open the can with the chilies in it and slice them up. Take out a bowl and mix together the eggs with half the cheese, the half and half, salt, and cumin.
2. Pour this mixture into a pan and then use some foil to cover it all up.
3. Add a trivet to the bottom of your slow cooker and then add this pan to the top of the trivet. Add in a cup of water to the slow cooker.
4. Place the lid on top of the slow cooker and then set it to the high temperature setting. After two hours, take the dish out and serve warm.

Overnight Breakfast Casserole

What's inside:

- Ground sausage (.5 lbs.)
- Chopped and cooked bacon (1 lb.)
- Cheddar cheese (2 c.)
- Mozzarella cheese (1 c.)
- Onion, diced (1)
- Green pepper, diced (1)
- Diced red pepper (1)
- Eggs (12)
- Almond milk (.5 c.)
- Salt (.5 tsp.)
- Pepper (.25 tsp.)
- Sweetener of choice (.25 tsp.)

How to make:

1. To start this recipe, take out the slow cooker and liberally grease the inside.
2. From here, add in half of your sausage, bacon, cheese, onion, green pepper, and red pepper. Repeat these layers until you have used up all of the ingredients above.
3. Take out a bowl and whisk together the eggs, milk, salt, pepper, and sweetener. Pour this on top of the layers of cheese.
4. Add the lid to the top of the slow cooker and pick the high temperature setting. After four hours, the dish is done and you can serve.

Mexican Breakfast Casserole

What's inside:

- Pork sausage roll (12 oz.)
- Garlic powder (.5 tsp.)
- Coriander (.5 tsp.)
- Cumin (1 tsp.)
- Chili powder (1 tsp.)
- Salt (.25 tsp.)
- Pepper (.25 tsp.)
- Salsa (1 c.)
- Almond milk (1 c.)
- Eggs (10)
- Pepper jack cheese (1 c.)

How to make:

1. Bring out a skillet and heat it up. Add in the pork and cook it up until all of the pink is gone. When the sausage is done, add in the seasonings and the salsa and combine well.
2. Bring out a bowl and whisk together the eggs and the milk. When those are combined together well, you can add the pork mixture to this and then stir in the cheese as well.
3. Take out the slow cooker and grease the bottom of it. Pour this mixture inside the slow cooker and then add the lid on top.
4. Turn on the slow cooker to the low setting and then cook for a bit. After five hours, you can take the dish out and top with some of your favorite toppings before serving.

Breakfast Pie

What's inside:

- Veggies of choice
- Whisked eggs (8)
- Shredded sweet potato (1)
- Pork breakfast sausage (1 lb.)
- Diced yellow onion (1)
- Garlic powder (1 Tbsp.)
- Dried basil (2 tsp.)

How to make:

1. Take out the slow cooker and grease the bottom of it up well.
2. Take out a shredder or another tool to help shred up the potato you will use.
3. Add the dried basil, garlic powder, yellow onion, breakfast sausage, sweet potato, whisked eggs, and other vegetables of choice.
4. Mix the ingredients around and then place the lid on top of the cooker. Turn it to a low setting.
5. After six to eight hours, the mixture should be done. You can slice it into eight slices and then serve.

Mushroom Melters

What's inside:

- Dried parsley (2 tsp.)
- Crushed garlic cloves (3)
- Brie (.3 lb. wheel)
- Mushrooms (12)

How to make:

1. Take out the slow cooker and drizzle a bit of olive inside. Lay the mushrooms out on a cutting board and then rub them with some olive oil.
2. Sprinkle the pepper, salt, herbs, and garlic all over the mushrooms and then place a piece of the brie on top of each mushroom.
3. Very carefully move the mushrooms over to the slow cooker, working to lay them out in a single layer.
4. Add the lid to the top of the slow cooker and then set the temperature to the high setting.
5. After 2 hours, the mushrooms will be done. Take out a skillet and heat up a bit of oil inside.
6. Move the cooked mushrooms to the skillet and cook them for just a minute or so to allow them to become golden on the bottom.
7. Serve on a platter with a sprinkling of grated parmesan cheese.

Hazelnut and Chocolate Pancakes

What's inside:

- Blueberries (.5 c.)
- Cinnamon (1 tsp.)
- Baking powder (.5 tsp.)
- Unsweetened cocoa powder (.25 c.)
- Ground hazelnuts (.5 c.)
- Eggs (2)
- Ricotta cheese (1 c.)

How to make:

1. Take out a bowl and mix together the cinnamon, salt, cocoa powder, ground hazelnuts, eggs, and ricotta cheese.
2. When those are mixed, add in the blueberries. Take out the slow cooker and add a bit of the coconut oil to the bottom.
3. Drop small dollops of this pancake mixture into the pot. It is fine if some of it runs together in the pot because you can separate it out when flipping later.
4. Place the lid on top of the slow cooker and then set the temperature to the highest setting.
5. After half an hour, open up the slow cooker and flip the pancakes around. Cook for another 30 minutes.
6. Serve with some berries, cream, or yogurt.

Cauliflower Breakfast Cake

What's inside:

- Chopped parsley
- Cheddar cheese (.5 c.)
- Sliced chorizo sausages (2)
- Sliced zucchini (2)
- Chopped red capsicums (2)
- Crushed garlic cloves (3)
- Cauliflower (.5 head)

How to make:

1. Take out a slow cooker and drizzle a bit of the olive oil inside. Add in the chorizo, zucchini, capsicums, cauliflower, and garlic inside.
2. Drizzle a bit of the olive oil in the slow cooker and then sprinkle the grated cheese over it all. Place the lid onto the slow cooker and then make sure that the temperature on a low setting.
3. After four hours, you can take the dish out of the slow cooker and then sprinkle on the fresh parsley before serving.

Keto Big Breakfast

What's inside:

- Lemon (1)
- Sliced avocadoes (2)
- Crumbled feta cheese (5 oz.)
- Red capsicum, sliced (1)
- Streaky bacon (8 slices)
- Beaten eggs (5)

How to make:

1. To start this recipe, take out the slow cooker and drizzle a bit of the olive oil inside.
2. When the slow cooker is set up, you can pour the egg into the pot and then add the pepper, salt, bacon, feta, and capsicum on top of the egg.
3. Add the lid to the top of the slow cooker and then set it up on the low setting.
4. After two hours, the cooking time is done. Take the dish out and slice it into four pieces.
5. Add the avocado slices on top and then drizzle with a bit of the olive oil. Add a squeeze of lemon juice on top before serving.

Chapter 10: Something on the Side – Easy Side Dishes

Garlic Brussel's Sprouts

What's inside:

- Lemon (.5)
- Cayenne pepper (.5 tsp.)
- Mayo (.5 c.)
- Dried chili flakes (1 tsp.)
- Crushed garlic cloves (3)
- Brussel's sprouts (16)

How to make:

1. Take out a skillet and drizzle a bit of olive oil in it to heat up. Once the oil has time to heat up, add in the sprouts and then toss around in the hot oil for a bit to make the outsides golden.
2. Place the prepared sprouts in your slow cooker and then sprinkle on the pepper, salt, chili flakes, and garlic on top.
3. Place the lid on the slow cooker and then set the heat so that it is at the low setting.
4. After two hours, with a chance to turn the sprouts over at one hour, the cooking is done.
5. Before serving, take out a small bowl and mix together the lemon juice, cayenne pepper, and mayo.
6. Take the sprouts out of the slow cooker and then serve with the mayo dip you just made.

Chicken and Bacon Teasers

What's inside:

- Streaky bacon (6 slices)
- Crushed garlic cloves (4)
- Grated cheddar cheese (.5 c.)
- Chicken breasts, sliced (2)

How to make:

1. Take out the slow cooker and coat it with some olive oil. Then take the pieces of chicken and wrap them up with the bacon. Add these into the slow cooker.
2. After these chicken and bacon pieces or organized, you can sprinkle on the crushed garlic, pepper, and salt on top.
3. Place the lid on the slow cooker and then set it to the low setting. Cook for about four hours on this setting.
4. After this time is up, you can take the chicken and bacon pieces out of the slow cooker. Arrange them inside an oven proof dish.
5. Turn on the oven and let it heat up to 350 degrees. Sprinkle some cheese on the chicken and then place in the oven so it has time to melt.
6. After the cheese is melted, take out of the oven and serve the teasers when they are hot.

Chive and Pork Meatballs

What's inside:

- Chives, chopped (2 Tbsp.)
- Ground almonds (.25 c.)
- Crushed garlic cloves (2)
- Egg (1)
- Minced pork (1 lb.)

How to make:

1. Take out a bit bowl and mix together the pepper, salt, chives, ground almonds, garlic, egg, and pork.
2. When this mixture is well combined, you can roll it into 18 balls. Then take out the slow cooker and drizzle a bit of olive oil inside of it.
3. Add the meatballs into the slow cooker and drizzle a bit of the olive oil on top. Add the lid on top of the pot and then set to the low setting.
4. After four hours, the meatballs should be done. You can take them out of the slow cooker and then serve warm.

Salmon Double Cheese Bites

What's inside:

- Lemon (1)
- Chopped spring onion (1)
- Mozzarella cheese, (.25 lbs. in 8 chunks)
- Firm cream cheese (.25 lb. in 8 chunks)
- Smoked salmon, sliced in half (4 strips)

How to make:

1. Take one of the cream cheese mixtures and one of the mozzarella pieces and press these together. Sprinkle with a bit of the spring onion.
2. Wrap these in the smoked salmon. Then repeat this process until you have eight of these balls ready to go.
3. Bring out your slow cooker and place the salmon bites into it, keeping them in one layer.
4. Place the lid on top of the pot and then set it at the lowest setting.
5. After 2 hours, the bites will be cooked through. You can then grate the zest from half the lemon and then place on a serving platter to enjoy.

Eggplant and Mini Lamb Skewer

What's inside:

- Chopped mint leaves (2 Tbsp.)
- Greek yogurt (.75 c.)
- Eggplant, sliced (1)
- Lemon (1)
- Crushed garlic cloves (2)
- Minced lamb (1 lb.)

How to make:

1. Take out a bowl and mix together the zest of one lemon, the pepper, salt, egg, garlic cloves, and minced lamb.
2. Roll this into 12 balls and set aside. Place the eggplant chunks on a towel and then sprinkle with some salt. Leave this to the side while you work on the yogurt dip.
3. Mix together the juice of the lemon, fresh mint, and yogurt in a bowl. Cover this up and then place the bowl in the fridge until you need it.
4. Rub the chunks of eggplant with some olive oil. Then bring out four skewers and fill them up, alternating between the lamb mince balls and the eggplant chunks. You want three of each on every skewer.
5. Take out the slow cooker and drizzle some olive oil inside. Lay these prepared skewers in the slow cooker and then set the temperature to a low setting.
6. After two hours, turn the skewers around and then place the lid back on for another two hours.
7. After this time, take the skewers out of the pot and then serve on a platter with the yogurt dip.

Spiced Macadamia and Chicken Nibbles

What's inside:

- Mixed paprika, cumin, and chili powder (2 tsp.)
- Salted and roasted macadamia nuts, chopped (.5 c.)
- Beaten eggs (2)
- Chicken nibbles (1.5 lbs.)

How to make:

1. To start this recipe, mix together the spices and chopped macadamia nuts. Take out another bowl and beat the egg inside..
2. Lightly coat each of the chicken pieces with the beaten egg, and the move right over to the plate of macadamia nuts and coat all around.
3. Bring out your slow cooker and drizzle some olive oil inside. Lay the chicken nibbles in a single layer inside.
4. Add the lid to the slow cooker and then set the temperature to a high setting. After two hours is done, the chicken can be taken out of the slow cooker.
5. Now you can bring out a skillet and heat up the olive oil. Move the chicken from the slow cooker and place into a hot skillet.
6. Fry both sides of the chicken until they are golden and crispy. Serve on a platter with your choice of dip and then serve.

Roasted Sweet Pepper Soup

What's inside:

- Sour cream (.5 c.)
- Ground coriander (1 tsp.)
- Cumin 1 tsp.)
- Stock cube, chicken (1)
- Chopped onion (1)
- Chopped garlic cloves (6)
- Chopped celery sticks (2)
- Chopped red capsicums (6)

How to make:

1. To start this recipe, take out the slow cooker and drizzle a bit of the olive oil inside.
2. When the slow cooker is set up, add in the pepper, salt, coriander, cumin, stock cube, onion, garlic, celery, capsicum, and two cups of water.
3. Add the lid to the top of the slow cooker and then make sure the temperature is set to low.
4. After six hours, you can turn off the heat. Use a hand held blender and blend your soup until it can become smooth.
5. Stir in the sour cream before you serve.

Rosemary and Lamb Stew

What's inside:

- Stock cube, lamb (1)
- Dried rosemary (2 tsp.)
- Chopped garlic cloves (4)
- Chopped onion (1)
- Lamb, cubed (2 lbs.)

How to make:

1. Take some olive oil and use it to drizzle the bottom of your slow cooker.
2. Take out a frying pan and add some oil to it as well. Brown the lamb in the frying pan for a few minutes.
3. Then add in the pepper, salt, stock cube, rosemary, garlic, and onion. Mix these together before adding to the slow cooker along with three cups of water.
4. Add the lid to the slow cooker and then make sure to set the temperature to a low setting.
5. After eight hours of cooking, stir this around and then serve while warm.

Coconut White Fish Soup

What's inside:

- Chopped coriander (1 handful) *or* parsley basil cilantro
- Lime (1)
- Coconut milk (3c.)
- Curry paste (2 Tbsp.)
- Grated ginger (2 tsp.)
- Chopped onion (1)
- Crushed garlic cloves (4)
- White fish, sliced (2 lbs.)

How to make:

1. Take out your slow cooker and drizzle a bit of olive oil inside to get it all set up and ready.
2. When the slow cooker is ready, add in half the coriander, juice from one lime, coconut milk, curry paste, ginger, onion, garlic, and fish. Stir this to combine.
3. When those are set up, place the lid on the pot and then turn the heat setting to low.
4. This will need to cook for five hours. After that time, take the lid from the slow cooker and then serve with the rest of the coriander on top.

Cheesy Broccoli and Leek Soup

What's inside:

- Full fat cream (1 c.)
- Grated cheddar cheese (1 c.)
- Chicken stock (2 c.)
- Garlic cloves, chopped (4)
- Sliced leek (1)
- Broccoli (1 head)

How to make:

1. Take out the slow cooker and drizzle in some of the olive oil inside.
2. Add the pepper, salt, stock, garlic, leek, and broccoli into the slow cooker and stir to combine.
3. Add the lid to the top of the slow cooker and then set the temperature setting to a high.
4. After this can cook for three hours, take the lid of the slow cooker, use a hand held blender to blend this soup until it is smooth.
5. Add the cream and cheese to the slow cooker and then stir around. Place the lid back on the slow cooker and turn the heat to high.
6. This can cook for another minute before serving.

Pumpkin and Parmesan Soup

What's inside:

- Heavy cream (.5 c.
- Parmesan cheese (.75 c.)
- Chicken stock (2 c.)
- Chopped garlic cloves (4)
- Chopped onion (1)
- Butternut pumpkin, cubed (1)

How to make:

1. To start this recipe, take out a slow cooker and then drizzle in some olive oil to prepare it.
2. Add the pepper, salt, stock, garlic, onion, and pumpkin to the slow cooker. Stir it around to combine.
3. Place the lid on the slow cooker and then set it to a high temperature. Cook this for about four hours.
4. When the time is over, take out the hand held blender and blend all of these ingredients together until they are smooth.
5. When those ingredients are smooth, you can stir the cream and the parmesan cheese. Leave the pot with the lid on for another twenty minutes to let the cheese melt all the way.
6. Serve while the mixture is hot.

Lettuce Beef Boats

What's inside:

- Pumpkin seeds (.25 c.)
- Grated Parmesan cheese (.5 c.)
- Crushed garlic cloves (2)
- Beef mince (1 lb.)
- Lettuce leaves (12)

How to make:

1. Take out the slow cooker and drizzle a bit of olive oil inside. Dd in the pepper, salt, parmesan, garlic, and beef mince.
2. Add the lid to the slow cooker and then turn the setting to a high.
3. After two hours, the beef should be cooked through, and the cheese should be melted.
4. Fill up each of the lettuce cups with a big spoon of this warm mince and then sprinkle on the pumpkin seeds on the top.
5. Serve these with a bit of olive and a sprinkling of salt and pepper.

Avocado, Cucumber, and Chicken Rolls

What's inside:

- Japanese mayo (3 Tbsp.)
- Sliced cucumber (.5)
- Sliced avocado (1)
- Nori sheets (3)
- Toasted sesame seeds (2 Tbsp.)
- Sesame oil (1 tsp.)
- Chicken breasts (3)

How to make:

1. Take out a slow cooker and then drizzle the olive oil inside. Add the chicken pieces to the slow cooker and then sprinkle the salt and pepper inside.
2. Pour the sesame seeds, sesame oil, and soy sauce over the chicken. Stir around to make sure that the chicken is coated.
3. Place the lid on top of the slow cooker and then set this to the low temperature.
4. After four hours, the chicken will be done.
5. At this time, you can prepare to make the rolls by making sure the cucumber and avocado is set up and ready, and the nori sheets laid out on a chopping board.
6. Place a row of the cooked chicken on the nori sheet, on the bottom third of it. Then place a row of avocado and a row of cucumber on top of the chicken.
7. If you are working with the Japanese mayo, place a thin line on top of the ingredients. Sprinkle on the sesame seeds on the filing.
8. Carefully roll up the nori with the filling tight inside. Seal up the edge with some water and then slice each one into eight pieces.
9. Serve this on a platter with some wasabi and soy sauce.

Mini Pumpkin Soups

What's inside:

- Heavy cream (.66 c.)
- Chicken stock (2 c.)
- Crushed garlic cloves (3)
- Chopped onion 1)
- Butternut pumpkin, chopped (2 lbs.)

How to make:

1. Take out the slow cooker and drizzle a bit of olive oil inside. Add in the pepper, salt, stock, garlic, onion, and pumpkin. Stir around to combine.
2. Add the lid to the top of the slow cooker and make sure the temperature is on high. Cook this for about three hours, or until the pumpkin has time to get soft.
3. Let this cool down a bit before using a hand-held blender to whiz the soup and make it smooth.
4. Stir the cream into the soup before adding in the pepper and salt. If you want to have a soup that is thinner, add in more cream.
5. Serve in some small serving mugs and enjoy.

Spiced Nut Snackers

What's inside:

- Curry powder (1 pinch)
- Salt (1 tsp.)
- Ground nutmeg (.5 tsp.)
- Cinnamon (2 tsp.)
- Melted coconut oil (2 Tbsp.)
- Melted butter (2 Tbsp.)
- Mixed nuts (4 c.)

How to make:

1. Take out the slow cooker and combine the curry powder, salt, nutmeg, cinnamon, coconut oil, and butter inside. Stir around to combine.
2. Add some of the nuts to the pot and then stir around until the nuts are completely coated. Add the lid to the top of the slow cooker and then set the temperature to a low.
3. After three hours, you can take the nuts out of the slow cooker. Serve these on a platter and then enjoy!

Cabbage and Chicken Dumplings

What's inside:

- Soy sauce (2 Tbsp.)
- Sesame oil (1 tsp.)
- Beaten egg (1)
- Chopped spring onion (1)
- Crushed garlic cloves (2)
- Shredded cabbage (2)
- Minced chicken (1 lb.)

How to make:

1. Take out a big bowl and add in the soy sauce, sesame oil, egg, spring onion, garlic, cabbage, and minced chicken. Mix together well.
2. Roll this mixture into 18 balls that are pretty even in size.
3. Take out the slow cooker and drizzle some oil inside. Lay the dumplings inside the pot and put into one layer if there is enough room.
4. Add the lid to the top of the slow cooker and set the temperature to low. After four hours, the dumplings should be done. Serve warm on a platter and enjoy.

Mini Lamb Burgers

What's inside:

- Cucumber slices (12)
- Mayo (.5 c.)
- Lettuce leaves (12)
- Slices cheddar cheese (12)
- Beaten egg (1)
- Dried herbs (1 tsp.)
- Crushed garlic cloves (3)
- Minced lamb (1 lb.)

How to make:

1. Take out a big bowl and combine together the pepper, salt, egg, dried herbs, garlic, and minced lamb together.
2. When this mixture is well combined, you can roll this into 12 balls and then flatten with your palm.
3. Drizzle some oil into your slow cooker and then add the lamb patties into the pot. Add a piece of cheese on top of the patty and then add the lid on top. Set this temperature to high.
4. After three hours, the patties can be done. Turn on the oven and let it heat up to 400 degrees on the grill setting.
5. Place these patties onto an oven tray and add into the oven as soon as it is warm enough.
6. Let these grill for a few minutes until you see the cheese is bubbling a bit and the patties are golden.
7. Assemble the burgers by placing a patty onto a lettuce leaf and then topping with the mayo, cucumber slices, and then fold the lettuce leave over before serving.

Chapter 11: Lunches for the Caveman in You

Beef Mince and Sausage Chili

What's inside:

- Sliced sausages (3)
- Dried chili flakes (1 tsp.)
- Smoked paprika (1 tsp.)
- Beef stock cubes (1)
- Chopped tomatoes (4)
- Crushed garlic cloves (4)
- Chopped onion (1)
- Minced beef (2 lbs.)

How to make:

1. To start this recipe, drizzle a bit of olive oil into the slow cooker.
2. When the slow cooker is prepared, add the pepper, salt, sausage, chili, paprika, stock cube, tomatoes, garlic, onion, minced beef, and one cup of water.
3. Place the lid onto your slow cooker and then turn the temperature to a low setting.
4. After eight hours of cooking, you can take the lid from the slow cooker, stir the chili, and then serve hot.

Lemon Butter Fish

What's inside:

- Chopped parsley (1 handful)
- Lemon (1)
- Crushed garlic cloves (2)
- Butter (2 oz.)
- White fish (6 fillets)

How to make:

1. Take out a bowl and combine together the pepper, salt, chopped parsley, zest from one lemon, garlic, and butter.
2. Prepare the slow cooker with some olive oil. Then add in the fish fillets into the slow cooker. Sprinkle with the pepper and salt.
3. Add a little bit of the lemon butter that we made before onto each fish fillet and then spread it all out.
4. Add the lid onto the slow cooker and then make sure the temperature is set to a low setting.
5. After five hours of cooking, the fish is done. Serve each fillet with some of the melted lemon butter and then serve.

Salmon and Garlic Greens

What's inside:

- Green beans (2 c.)
- Sliced broccoli (.5 head)
- Crushed garlic cloves (4)
- Salmon fillets (4)

How to make:

1. Take out the slow cooker and prepare it with some olive oil inside.
2. When the slow cooker is set up, place the salmon fillet into the pot and then sprinkle on some pepper and salt.
3. Now add the garlic, beans, and broccoli on top of the salmon, and sprinkle all of this with the pepper and salt.
4. Drizzle some more of the olive oil on top of the fish and the vegetables.
5. Add the lid onto the slow cooker and then turn the heat up to a high temperature.
6. This can cook for about three hours. Check the fish to make sure it is done before serving right away.

Coconut Fish Curry

What's inside:

- Coriander
- Lime (1)
- Coconut milk (2 cans)
- Fish stock (2 c.)
- Yellow curry paste (2 Tbsp.)
- Turmeric (1 tsp.)
- Chopped onion (1)
- Crushed garlic cloves (4)
- White fish (4)

How to make:

1. Take out the slow cooker and get it all set up with some olive oil.
2. Add the pepper, salt, coconut milk, stock, fish, curry paste, turmeric, onion, and garlic into the slow cooker, taking the time to stir around to combine.
3. Add the lid onto the slow cooker and then set the temperature to a high setting.
4. After four hours of cooking, you can serve the fish dish hot with a bit of lime juice and coriander on top.

Bacon and Fish Soup

What's inside:

- Crème fraiche (1 c.)
- Fish stock (4 c.)
- Crushed garlic cloves (5)
- Chopped white fish (4 fillets)
- Chopped streaky bacon (5 slices)

How to make:

1. Take out the slow cooker and make sure that it is set up with some olive oil inside.
2. When the slow cooker is ready, you can add the pepper, salt, stock, garlic, fish, and bacon inside.
3. Add the lid to the slow cooker and make sure that the temperature is set to a high setting.
4. This dish will need to cook for about four hours. When that four hours is over, you can remove the lid and then slowly stir the crème fraiche into the soup.
5. Stir this around and then serve while hot.

Mozzarella Shrimp Parcels

What's inside:

- Small skewers (12)
- Kale (1 bunch)
- Mozzarella cheese (2 c.)
- Streaky bacon (12 slices)
- Frozen shrimp (2 c.)

How to make:

1. To start this recipe, you would cut the kale into 12 large pieces. Ten take out a large board and lay out the kale on it.
2. Lay two bacon half slices on the kale and then top with a bit of the shrimp on top of that.
3. Top the bacon and shrimp with some of the grated mozzarella. Sprinkle with some pepper and salt.
4. When all of these are connected together, you can wrap the parcels p tightly by folding up the sides, then folding the top and bottom up, and then use a skewer to secure them.
5. Take out the slow cooker and prepare it with some of the olive oil. Add the parcels into the slow cooker when it is all set up.
6. Add the lid on top of the slow cooker and then turn the heat setting to high. After three hours, the dish is done.
7. Once the cooking time is done, add a bit of olive oil into a frying pan. Take the parcels out of your slow cooker and then move them to the hot olive oil to cook on both sides.
8. Serve with some dips and sauces and enjoy.

Salsa and Cheese Chicken

What's inside:

- Chicken (1.5 lbs.)
- Salsa (1.5 c.)
- Shredded cheese (1.5 c.)

How to make:

1. Take out the slow cooker and use some olive oil to grease your slow cooker.
2. Add the chicken to the slow cooker and then top with some salsa. Add the lid to the slow cooker.
3. Cook this on a high setting for a bit. After 2 hours of cooking, you can turn the slow cooker off.
4. Turn on the oven and give it some time to turn up to 425 degrees. Add the chicken to a greased sheet.
5. Use the salsa from the pot to help cover the chicken and then top with some cheese. Add this to the oven to bake.
6. After 15 minutes, take the chicken out and garnish with some cilantro and sour cream before serving.

Taco Turkey Lettuce Wraps

What's inside:

- Ground turkey (1 lb.)
- Chopped onion (.5 c.)
- Garlic cloves (2)
- Chili powder (2 Tbsp.)
- Cumin (.5 tsp.)
- Tomato sauce (8 oz.)
- Red pepper (.5 tsp.)
- Chicken broth (.5 c.)

How to make:

1. Add the ground turkey to a skillet and cook it through until all the pink is gone.
2. Take out a bowl and add the ground turkey, red pepper, tomato sauce, cumin, chili powder, garlic cloves, and chopped onion inside. Stir around to incorporate well.
3. Pour this mix into your prepared slow cooker and then place the lid on top of theecooker.
4. Turn this on to a low setting and let the mixture cook. After six hours, turn the slow cooker off.
5. Lay the lettuce leaves out on the counter and top with some of the ground turkey mixture that is in the slow cooker.
6. Wrap the lettuce up around the filling and then serve.

Shrimp Fajitas

What's inside:

- Sliced green pepper (2)
- Sliced red peppers (2)
- Quartered tomato (1)
- Sliced onion (1)
- Shrimp (1 lb.)
- Chicken broth (.5 c.)
- Taco seasoning (1 packet)
- Chili powder (1 tsp.)
- Paprika (.5 tsp.)
- Salt (1 tsp.)

How to make:

1. Take out the slow cooker and set it up with a bit of olive oil in the bottom.
2. When the slow cooker is ready, add the green peppers, red peppers, tomato, onion, chicken broth, taco seasoning, chili powder, paprika, and salt.
3. Place the lid on top and cook this on a low setting. After two hours, take the lid off the slow cooker and add the shrimp on top.
4. Turn the heat up to high and let it cook for another half an hour or so to get the shrimp cooked through. Serve warm.

Steak Bites

What's inside:

- Round steak (4 lbs.)
- Beef broth (.5 c.)
- Minced onion (1 Tbsp.)
- Garlic powder (1 tsp.)
- Salt (.5 tsp.)
- Pepper (.5 tsp.)
- Butter (4 Tbsp.)

How to make:

1. Take the steak and cut it into small cubes. Add the cubes into your slow cooker and pour some of the broth on top.
2. From here, sprinkle the meat with the onion, garlic powder, pepper. Slice up the butter and then place on top of everything.
3. Place the lid on top of the slow cooker and cook on a low setting. After six hours, you can take the meal out of the slow cooker and serve.

Pork Carnitas

What's inside:

- Pork chops (3 lbs.)
- Diced onion (1)
- Sliced yellow pepper (1)
- Sliced orange pepper (1)
- Sliced red pepper (1)
- Minced garlic cloves (2)
- Chili powder (2 Tbsp.)
- Cumin (1 Tbsp.)
- Bay leaves (2)
- Taco sauce (.5 c.)
- Water (.5 c.)

How to make:

1. To start this recipe, take out the slow cooker and add the water inside before adding in the pork chops as well.
2. Add the taco sauce, bay leaves, cumin, chili powder, minced garlic cloves, sliced red pepper, orange pepper, yellow pepper, and diced onion. Stir these together well to combine.
3. Place the lid on top of the slow cooker and then set to a low setting for about 8 hours to cook.
4. After this time is up, you can take the meat out and use some forks to shred up the meat. Serve this warm.

Pork Chops

What's inside:

- Heavy cream (1 c.)
- Chopped mushrooms (2 c.)
- Dried herbs, mixed (1 tsp.)
- Chopped onion (1)
- Chopped garlic cloves (4)
- Pork chops (6)

How to make:

1. Take the pork chops and rub them all over with the olive oil, pepper, and salt. Take out a frying pan and heat up some oil inside.
2. When the oil is hot, add in the mushrooms, onion, and garlic. Cook these until they are hot. Add in the cream to the pan and let it simmer for a bit to reduce slightly.
3. Take out the slow cooker and prepare it with some of the olive oil. Add in the pork chops to the slow cooker and ten pour the cream of mushroom mixture on top.
4. Top all of this with the pepper, salt, and mixed dried herbs. Add the lid onto the pot and then set the time to a high temperature.
5. Cook this mixture for about four hours. When you are ready to serve, make sure that the dish is hot and top with a spoonful of creamy mushroom sauce over the top.

Paprika drumsticks

What's inside:

- Ground almond (.25 c.)
- Beaten eggs (2)
- Smoky paprika (2 tsp.)
- Chicken drumsticks (10)

How to make:

1. Take out a plate and mix together the pepper, salt, ground almond, and paprika. In another bowl, you can add the egg into it.
2. Prepare the chicken drumsticks by dipping them in the beaten egg and then rolling them through the paprika and almond mixture that you already made.
3. Take out your slow cooker and drizzle a bit of olive inside of it.
4. Place the drumsticks into the slow cooker and then add the lid on top. Turn this on to the high temperature setting.
5. This dish will need to cook for about four hours. When the chicken is done, serve with a nice salad and enjoy.

Beef Pot Roast

What's inside:

- Dried herbs (1 tsp.)
- Beef stock (1 c.)
- Dijon mustard (1 Tbsp.)
- Garlic cloves (6)
- Onions (2)
- Beef roast (4 lbs.)

How to make:

1. Take out a frying pan and heat up some oil inside. Once the oil is nice and warm, you can sear the beef roast on all sides until it becomes browned.
2. Prepare the slow cooker with some olive oil and then add the garlic and onions inside the pot.
3. In another bowl, mix together the herbs, beef stock, and Dijon mustard.
4. Add the beef into your slow cooker and then top with the onions. Rub the beef with the salt and the pepper.
5. Pour the stock and mustard mixture on top of the beef and then place the lid on top of this.
6. Make sure that the slow cooker is turned to the high temperature to cook the pot roast.
7. After six hours the dish will be done. Remove the beef from the pot and then let it rest and cool down a bit before carving and enjoying.

Tuna Steaks

What's inside:

- White wine (.5 c.)
- Sliced lemon (1)
- Crushed garlic cloves (3)
- Tuna steaks (4)

How to make:

1. Take out a pot and add the white wine into it. You want to reduce this by simmering until the smell of alcohol has cooked off.
2. Rub the tuna steaks with the olive oil and sprinkle on with some of the pepper and salt. Then add this tuna steak into the slow cooker.
3. Sprinkle a bit of the crushed garlic on top of the tuna steaks. Add two lemon slices on top of each steak and then pour the reduced wine into the pot.
4. Add the lid to the top of the slow cooker and then set this to a high temperature setting.
5. After three hours of cooking, the tuna steaks will be done. Serve this with a bit of the liquid that is leftover in the slow cooker, and a side salad.

Spinach and Chicken Stew

What's inside:

- Heavy cream (.5 c.)
- Dry white wine (.5 c.)
- Chicken stock (2 c.)
- Dried tarragon (1 tsp.)
- Crushed garlic cloves (6)
- Chopped onion (1)
- Chopped spinach (2 c.)
- Chicken thighs (2 lbs.)

How to make:

1. Take out the slow cooker and add in the pepper, salt, tarragon, stock, garlic cloves, onion, spinach, and chicken.
2. Place the lid on top of the slow cooker and then set the temperature to be low. Let these cook together for a bit.
3. After eight hours, take out a small pot and drizzle a bit of olive oil inside. Add in the wine and a few garlic cloves. . Let this simmer until it is reduced.
4. Add the cream to the pot that has the wine and then stir the ingredients around to combine.
5. Take the lid off the slow cooker and then stir the cream and wine mixture inside. Serve while warm.

Layered Cheeseburger Stew

What's inside:

- Mustard for serving
- Mayo for serving
- Sliced tomato (1)
- Chopped iceberg lettuce (.5 head)
- Grated cheddar cheese (2 c.)
- Sliced pickles (.25 c.)
- Chopped tomatoes (2)
- Beef stock cube (1)
- Chopped onion (1)
- Minced beef (2 lbs.)

How to make:

1. Bring out the slow cooker and then add in a cup of water along with the pepper, salt, tinned tomatoes, stock cube, garlic, onion, and minced beef. Stir around to combine.
2. Add the lid to the top of the slow cooker and then let the temperature get to a high setting.
3. After four hours of cooking, take the lid off of the slow cooker and place a layer of pickles on top of it all along with a layer of cheese.
4. Add the lid back to the slow cooker and cook on the high setting. After another half an hour, serve with some of the mustard, mayo, tomato, and lettuce.

Chapter 12: Dinners That Will Have Your Family Begging for More

Meat Lover's Pizza

What's inside:

- Dried oregano (1 tsp.)
- Grated cheddar cheese (.5 c.)
- Grated mozzarella cheese (1 c.)
- Tomato puree (.5 c.)
- Capsicum, green (1)
- Pepperoni (18 slices (
- Parmesan cheese, grated (.5 c.)
- Beaten egg (1)
- Cauliflower (.5 head)

How to make:

1. Take out a bowl and then mix together the pepper, salt, parmesan, egg, and blitzed cauliflower. Mix this until you get a type of dough to form.
2. Take out the slow cooker and drizzle some olive oil inside. When the slow cooker is prepared, you can press the cauliflower mixture inside of it.
3. Spread the tomato puree over this base and then sprinkle the mozzarella and cheddar on top of it all.
4. Then to this with the pepperoni slices and sprinkle the oregano over the meat slices.
5. Add the lid to the top of the slow cooker and make sure the temperature is on a high setting.
6. After four hours, you can turn off the slow cooker and then serve a slice of this with any other keto approved sides you would like.

Beef and Veggie Stew

What's inside:

- Cubed beef sirloin tip (2 lbs.)
- Olive oil (2 Tbsp.)
- Chopped baby carrots (1 lb.)
- Chopped yellow onions (1 lb.)
- Quartered white button mushrooms (6 oz.)
- Dry white wine (1 c.)
- Sliced celery stalks (6)
- Minced garlic cloves (6)
- Tomato paste (.25 c.)
- Bay leaves (2)
- Minced thyme leaves (2 tsp.)
- Pepper (1 tsp.)
- Salt (1.5 tsp.)
- Honeyville almond flour (.33 c.)
- Beef broth (5 c.)
- Sliced cauliflower (1 head)

How to make:

1. Take out a pan and heat up some oil inside. Once the oil is warmed up, sear the cubes of beef until they are browned. Set these to the side.
2. When the beef is done, add the onions to the same pan and cook for a few minutes until it is fragrant.
3. Bring out the slow cooker and prepare with a bit of butter and olive oil. Add in the onions and beef to the slow cooker along with the rest of the ingredients. Season with the salt and pepper.
4. Place the lid on top of the slow cooker and then set on a low temperature. After 8 hours, you can serve this stew with some sour cream and enjoy.

Cuban Mojo Pork

What's inside:

- Pork shoulder (1)
- Salt (1.5 tsp.)
- Pepper (1 tsp.)
- Orange juice (.75 c.)
- Lime juice (.5 c.)
- Zest from one orange
- Zest from one lime
- Olive oil (.5 c.)
- Garlic cloves (8)
- Oregano (2 tsp.)
- Cumin (2 tsp.)
- Chopped cilantro (.25 c.)

How to make:

1. Take the pork and lay it out on the table. Make a few slits in it using your knife.
2. Add the pork along with the rest of the ingredients into the slow cooker and then mix it all around well. Make sure to ladle the liquids on top of the pork.
3. Add the lid to the slow cooker and then turn it onto the high setting. Cook this for about five hours.
4. After this time, you can take the pork out of the slow cooker and then add it to a sheet that is lined with foil.
5. Turn on the oven and let it have time to heat up to 400 degrees. Take the pork and place it into the oven to bake.
6. After 15 minutes, the pork is done and you can take it out and serve sliced up and warm.

Mexican Meatloaf

What's inside:

- Ground beef (1 lb.)
- Ground turkey (1 lb.)
- Egg (1)
- Sour cream (.33 c.)
- Chopped green chilies (4.5 oz.)
- Onion (1)
- Taco seasoning packet (1)
- Red bell pepper (1)
- Carrot (1)
- Celery stalk (1)
- Enchilada sauce (19 oz.)
- Shredded cheese (1 c.)

How to make:

1. To start, take out a big bowl and add both of the ground meats inside. When those are well combined, add in the egg, sour cream, and taco seasoning.
2. Trim the vegetables and then add them to your food processor. Process these until they are smooth and then pour the vegetable mixture into the bowl.
3. Use your hands to mix up all of these ingredients until they are combined. Shape this into a log or into a shape that works for your slow cooker.
4. Add this to the slow cooker and pour the sauce on top. Place the lid on the slow cooker and set it to the low temperature.
5. After six hours, you can sprinkle the cheese on top right before serving.

Seafood Gumbo

What's inside:

- Sliced sea bass fillets (24 oz.)
- Ghee (3 Tbsp.)
- Cajun seasoning (3 Tbsp.)
- Diced yellow onion (2)
- Diced bell peppers (2)
- Diced celery ribs (4)
- Diced tomatoes (28 oz.)
- Tomato paste (.25 c.)
- Bay leaves (3)
- Bone broth (1.5 c.)
- Raw shrimp (2 lbs.)

How to make:

1. Take the fillets and then use the pepper and salt to season them. Add half of the Cajun seasoning on top.
2. Place the ghee into a skillet and then once the ghee is warm, add the fillet chunks to it. Cook these for a few minutes on all sides.
3. After this time, you can add the onions, pepper, celery, and Cajun seasoning. Cook for a few more minutes until fragrant.
4. Prepare the slow cooker and then add the cooked fish, diced tomatoes, tomato paste, bay leaves, or broth. Mix all of these ingredients together well.
5. Place the lid on the slow cooker and set it to the low temperature. After seven hours, turn the slow cooker off and serve warm.

Tilapia with Roasted Pepper Sauce

What's inside:

- Tilapia fillets (1 lb.)
- Butter (3 Tbsp.)
- Diced onion (1)
- Chopped garlic cloves (2)
- Chopped roasted peppers (6 oz.)
- Roasted peppers (6 oz.)
- Heavy cream (.75 c.)
- Grated Parmesan cheese (.5 c.)

How to make:

1. Bring out a skillet and warm up a few tablespoons of butter inside. Warm this up and then add the tilapia fillets. Cook this for a few minutes to get the fish cooked all the way through.
2. When those are cooked, use the salt and pepper to season the fillets and then set it to the side.
3. In the same skillet, add the diced onion inside along with the butter. Cook for about five more minutes.
4. At this time, add the garlic to this onion along with the pureed and chopped roasted peppers. Cook this for a bit longer to make soft and warm.
5. Now you can add in the heavy cream and parmesan cheese. Take the skillet from the heat, stir, and adjust the seasoning if it is needed.
6. Take out your slow cooker and prepare it. Add all of the ingredients from the skillet to the slow cooker and put the lid on top.
7. Cook this for about an hour. After that time, garnish the dish with some parsley and a bit more parmesan cheese and then serve warm.

Beef Shank

What's inside:

- Rosemary sprig (1)
- Beef stock (3 c.)
- Red wine (2 c.)
- Chopped garlic cloves (5)
- Chopped onion (1)
- Beef shanks (2 lbs.)

How to make:

1. Take out a frying pan and heat up a bit of olive oil inside. When this is warm, add the beef shanks and then brown to help seal it on each side.
2. Take the beef shanks out and then set aside. Add the wine into the skillet and then simmer a bit to reduce.
3. Prepare your slow cooker with some olive oil before adding in the pepper, salt, rosemary, stock, reduced wine, garlic, onion, and beef shanks.
4. Place the lid on top of the slow cooker and set the temperature to a low setting.
5. After 8 hours, check the meat. If it is tender, then you can serve it with a side of vegetables.

Stuffed Chicken Breasts

What's inside:

- Mozzarella cheese (.5 c.)
- Mixed herbs, dried (.5 tsp.)
- Chopped tomatoes (2)
- Chopped baby spinach (1 c.)
- Chopped black olives (12)
- Sliced mozzarella cheese (.5 lbs.)
- Chopped garlic cloves (4)
- Chicken breasts (4)

How to make:

1. Take the chicken and slice them going lengthwise, so that the cavity can open but the two pieces are still connected together.
2. Rub the chicken with some olive oil and then sprinkle on the pepper and salt.
3. Stuff each breast with the spinach, olive, mozzarella, and garlic. Add the chicken to the slow cooker and pour the tomatoes on top. Make sure to sprinkle on the mixed herbs over it all.
4. Turn the temperature on to a high setting and place the lid on the top. After four hours, you can take the lid off and sprinkle on the extra cheese.
5. Cook a bit longer so that the cheese can melt before serving hot.

Beef Lasagna

What's inside:

- Ricotta cheese (1 c.)
- Mozzarella cheese (1 c.)
- Cheese (2 c.)
- Chopped tomatoes (4)
- Baby spinach (2 c.)
- Sliced zucchinis (2)
- Sliced eggplant (1)
- Dried mixed herbs (2 tsp)
- Chopped garlic cloves (5)
- Chopped onion (1)
- Minced beef (2 lbs.)

How to make:

1. Bring out a frying pan with deep sides and heat up a bit of olive oil inside. When the oil is warm, add in the garlic and the onions and then cook until they are soft.
2. At this time, add in the minced beef and cook a bit to begin the browning process. Add in the mixed herbs and tomatoes and sprinkle with the pepper and salt. Cook for another five minutes.
3. Set up the slow cooker with some olive oil. Spread a layer of beef mixture into the pot, add a layer of eggplant, and then another layer of the beef mixture on top of this.
4. Now add in a layer of zucchini, another of beef, a layer of spinach, and then the rest of the beef mixture on top of the spinach mixture.
5. Take out a big bowl and mix together the pepper, salt, ricotta cheese, mozzarella cheese, and cheddar cheese.
6. Spread this mixture all over the lasagna and then add the lid to the top. Set the temperature to the high setting.
7. After four hours, the dish is done and you can serve while it is hot.

Lamb Curry

What's inside:

- Greek yogurt
- Chopped coriander
- Chopped tomatoes (2)
- Coconut milk (2.5)
- Lamb stock cube (1)
- Curry paste (4 Tbsp.)
- Chopped garlic cloves (5)
- Chopped onions (2)
- Boneless lamb (2.5 lbs.)

How to make:

1. Take out a pan and heat up some oil inside. Add the lamb to the hot pan and then cook it long enough to seal on all sides, which can take three minutes.
2. Prepare your slow cooker with some olive oil before adding the lamb, pepper, salt, curry paste, garlic, and onions in the pot. Stir to coat the lamb in the curry paste.
3. From here, you can add in a cup of water, the chopped tomatoes, stock cube, and coconut milk to the slow cooker.
4. Add the lid to the top of the slow cooker and then set this to a low setting. After eight hours, the dish is done and you can serve with some coriander on top and a side of Greek yogurt.

Butter Chicken

What's inside:

- Heavy cream (.5 c.)
- Butter (3 Tbsp.)
- Chopped tomatoes (2)
- Tomato paste (2 Tbsp.)
- Greek yogurt (.5 c.)
- Chili powder (2 tsp.)
- Garam Masala (2 Tbsp.)
- Chopped coriander (1 handful)
- Grated ginger (2 Tbsp.)
- Chopped onion (1)
- Crushed garlic cloves (6)
- Boneless chicken thigh (2 lbs.)

How to make:

1. Take out a bit bowl and add together the pepper, salt, yogurt, tomato paste, coriander, ginger, onion, garlic, and chicken thighs. Stir this to combine and to make sure that the chicken is coated all the way through.
2. Let the chicken marinate in this for at least four hours. If you can do this the night before, it is even better.
3. When you are ready to make the meal, take out the slow cooker and then drizzle in a bit of olive oil.
4. Add the chili powder and the Garam Masala to the slow cooker to create a paste and then add in the chicken and marinade to the pot and stir around.
5. From here, add in the pepper, salt, butter, and tomatoes. Add the lid on top of the slow cooker and set it to a low temperature.
6. Let this cook for eight hours. After this time, take the lid off and stir the cream into this before serving.

Whole Chicken for Dinner

What's inside:

- Butter (3 Tbsp.)
- Chicken stock (.75 c.)
- Celery sticks (3)
- Onions, sliced (2)
- Garlic cloves (6)
- Lemon (1)
- Dried herbs (1 tsp.)
- Chicken, whole (1)

How to make:

1. To start this recipe, take out a slow cooker and prepare it with the olive oil.
2. You can then prepare the chicken. Do this by rubbing it all over with some olive oil and then sprinkling the pepper, salt, and dried herbs all over it. Stuff the lemon into the cavity of the chicken.
3. From here, you can add the garlic cloves, celery chunks, and onion chunks to the slow cooker and top with some of the stock. Lay the chicken over it all.
4. Make sure to add a knob of butter to the top of the chicken and press it down into the chicken.
5. Add the lid on top of the slow cooker and then turn it to the high temperature setting.
6. This dish needs to cook for six hours. After this time, take the lid off and remove the chicken. Let the other ingredients cool down a bit before serving.

Pork Roast

What's inside:

- Chopped fresh herbs
- Chicken stock (1 c.)
- Chunked onions (2)
- Pork shoulder (5 lbs.)

How to make:

1. Take out a frying pan and heat up a bit of oil inside. When the oil is nice and warm, add the pork shoulder in, with the fat side down, and then sear the fat for a bit.
2. Then work on searing all the sides of the pork until it is turned browned.
3. Take out the slow cooker and prepare it with some olive oil. Add the onion chunks on the bottom of the prepared slow cooker and then pour the chicken stock over it.
4. When those are prepared, place the pork shoulder on top of the onions. Rub the pork skin with some herbs, pepper, and salt and then add the lid on top of the slow cooker.
5. Set the temperature of the slow cooker to a low setting. Cook this for eight hours and then serve warm.

Stuffed Beef Packets

What's inside:

- Wooden skewers, in half (3)
- Pine nuts (3 Tbsp.)
- Chopped black olives (18)
- Chopped baby spinach (1 c.)
- Ricotta cheese (1 c.)
- Feta cheese (4 oz.)
- Beef schnitzel (6 slices)

How to make:

1. To start this recipe, take out a small bowl and mix together the pepper, salt, pine nuts, olives, spinach, ricotta cheese, and feta cheese.
2. When those are combined, take each of your beef schnitzel slices and lay them out on a board. Place a bit of the cheese mixture into the middle of each one.
3. Grab the sides of the schnitzel around the filling and wrap them up tightly. Use the halves of the skewers in order to secure the packets. Sprinkle the top with some pepper and salt.
4. Bring out the slow cooker and prepare it with some olive oil drizzled around inside. Set the temperature of the slow cooker to high.
5. Place the beef packets into the slow cooker and place the lid on top. After four hours of cooking, these beef packets should be done.
6. Give them some time to cool and then serve with either a side of relish or another sauce that is keto friendly.

Salmon Cake

What's inside:

- Coriander (1 handful)
- Smoked salmon (1 fillet)
- Baby spinach, chopped (1 c.)
- Heavy cream (3 Tbsp.)
- Beaten eggs (4)

How to make:

1. Take out the slow cooker and prepare it with some olive oil inside.
2. After the slow cooker is done, you can add in the pepper, salt, salmon, spinach, cream, and beaten egg inside.
3. After stirring, place the lid onto the slow cooker and then make sure that the temperature is set to a low setting.
4. This dish can cook for the next four hours. When that is done, check to make sure that the salmon and the eggs are cooked through.
5. Serve this dish with a good sprinkling of fresh coriander.

Sausage and Prawn Slow Cooker Casserole

What's inside:

- Mixed dried spices (2 tsp.)
- Mixed dried herbs (1 tsp.)
- Chopped tomatoes(4)
- Chopped onion (1)
- Crushed garlic cloves (5)
- Chopped sausages (3)
- Frozen prawns (1.5 c.)

How to make:

1. To start this recipe, take out the slow cooker and drizzle a bit of olive oil inside.
2. When the slow cooker is ready, add the pepper, salt, spices, herbs, tomatoes, onion, garlic, sausages, and prawns into it.
3. Add the lid into the pot and then make sure that the temperature is set to a low setting.
4. This dish needs to cook for about six hours. When the dish is done, you can serve hot with some fresh herbs on top.

Chapter 13: Tasty Desserts

Keto Hot Chocolate

How to make:

- Stevia to taste
- Cinnamon (.5 tsp.)
- Dark chocolate, chopped (3 oz.)
- Cocoa powder (.33 c.)
- Vanilla (1 tsp.)
- Heavy cream (2 c.)
- Coconut milk (5 c.)

How to make:

1. Take out your slow cooker and add in the stevia, cinnamon, chocolate, cocoa powder, vanilla, cream, and coconut milk. Stir these around to combine.
2. Place a lid on top of the slow cooker and set the temperature to the high setting.
3. During the cooking process, make sure to whisk the mixture every 45 minutes. After four hours, the chocolate should be done.
4. Pour into your favorite glass and enjoy some whipped cream on top.

Blueberry Lemon Custard Cake

What's inside:

- Eggs, separated(6)
- Almond flour (.5 c.)
- Lemon zest (2 tsp.)
- Lemon stevia (1 tsp.)
- Sweetener of choice (.5 c.)
- Salt (.5 tsp.)
- Light cream (2 c.)
- Blueberries (.5 c.)

How to make:

1. Take out your mixer and add in the egg whites. You will want to whip these until you get some soft peaks to form. Set these to the side.
2. Whisk the yolks in with the rest of the ingredients, except for the blueberries. Slowly fold in the egg whites at this time.
3. Bring out your slow cooker and grease it with a bit of butter. Pour the batter inside and then sprinkle on the blueberries.
4. Place the lid on top and set this to cook on a low setting for an hour.
5. Place into the fridge after this time and let it chill for a minimum of two hours, or overnight, before serving.

Keto Chocolate Cake

What's inside:

- Almond flour (1 c. and 2 Tbsp.)
- Swerve (.5 c.)
- Cocoa powder (.5 c.)
- Whey protein powder (3 Tbsp.)
- Baking powder (1.5 tsp.)
- Salt (.25 tsp.)
- Eggs (3)
- Melted butter (6 Tbsp.)
- Unsweetened almond milk (.66 c.)
- Vanilla (.75 tsp.)
- Chocolate chips, sugar free (.33 c.)

How to make:

1. To begin this recipe, use some butter to prepare the slow cooker.
2. Take out a bowl and mix together the flour, sweetener, cocoa powder, protein powder, baking powder, and salt.
3. After this time, mix in the butter, eggs, almond milk, and vanilla. Once those are prepared, you can fold in the chocolate chips.
4. Pour the whole mixture into the prepared slow cooker and then add the lid on top. Set this to the low setting.
5. After 2 and a half hours, turn the slow cooker off and let them cool down. Slice this into pieces and serve.

Lemon Crock Pot Cake

What's inside:

- Honeyville almond flour (1.5 c.)
- Coconut flour (.5 c.)
- Swerve sweetener (3 Tbsp.)
- Baking powder (2 tsp.)
- Xanthan gum (.5 tsp.)
- Melted butter (.5 c.)
- Whipping cream (.5 c.)
- Lemon juice (2 Tbsp.)
- Zest from two lemons
- Eggs (2)
- *Topping*
- Swerve sweetener (3 Tbsp.)
- Boiling water (.5 c.)
- Melted butter (2 Tbsp.)
- Lemon juice (2 Tbsp.)

How to make:

1. Bring out a bowl and combine together the flour, sweetener, baking powder, and xanthan gum.
2. In another bowl, whisk together the butter, whipping cream, lemon juice and zest, and egg.
3. When those two bowls are done, combine them together until they are well incorporated. Pour the whole batter mix into a greased slow cooker.
4. To make the topping, combine together the lemon juice, melted butter, boiling water, and swerve sweetener together. Spread this on top of the cake mixture already in the slow cooker.
5. Place the lid on top of the slow cooker and set it to the high temperature setting.
6. After three hours of cooking, turn the slow cooker off and serve warm with some fresh fruit and whipped cream.

Pumpkin Custard

What's inside:

- Eggs (4)
- Granulated stevia (.5 c.)
- Pumpkin puree (1 c.)
- Vanilla (1 tsp.)
- Honeyville almond flour (.5 c.)
- Pumpkin pie spice (1 tsp.)
- Salt (.25 tsp.)
- Butter (4 Tbsp.)

How to make:

1. Take out the slow cooker to start up this recipe and grease it with some butter.
2. Bring out a bowl and beat the eggs until it is smooth. Then beat in the sweetener slowly. Add in the pumpkin puree and vanilla until these are blended together well.
3. At this time, add in the almond flour, salt, and pumpkin pie spice. Blend this as you add in the butter.
4. Pour this mixture into the slow cooker. Place a paper towel over the opening of the pot before you close it.
5. Turn this to a low setting and let it cook for about 2 to 2 and a half hours.
6. When you are ready to serve, add some whipped cream and a dash of nutmeg on top.

Blackberry and Chocolate Chip Cake

What's inside:

- Honeyville almond flour (2 c.)
- Shredded coconut (1 c.)
- Swerve sweetener (.5)
- Chocolate whey protein powder (.25 c.)
- Baking soda (2 tsp.)
- Salt (.25 tsp.)
- Eggs (4)
- Melted coconut oil (.25 c.)
- Melted butter (.25 c.)
- Heavy cream (.5 c.)
- Blackberries (1 c.)
- Dark chocolate chips, sugar free (.33 c.)

How to make:

1. Take out the slow cooker and use some butter to grease up the inside of the pot.
2. Inside one bowl, add in all of the dry ingredients and mix them together. Add in all of the wet ingredients, making sure that it is all blended together well.
3. Pour the batter into a prepared slow cooker. Add the lid to the slow cooker and make it be on the low setting.
4. After three hours the dish is done. You can serve with some blackberries on top and then serve.

Ambrosia

What's inside:

- Fresh berries (1 c.)
- Greek yogurt (2 c.)
- Heavy cream (2 c.)
- Cinnamon (1 tsp.)
- Salted butter (2 oz.)
- Pumpkin seeds (.33 c.)
- Dark chocolate (3 oz.)
- Slivered almonds (.75 c.)
- Shredded coconut (1 c.)

How to make:

1. Take out your slow cooker and set it all up. Add the cinnamon, butter, pumpkin seeds, dark chocolate, slivered almonds, and shredded coconut inside.
2. When those are all well mixed, add the lid to the slow cooker and set it to a high setting.
3. After three hours, with some stirring every 45 minutes, you can remove the mixture from the slow cooker and set it in a bowl to cool down.
4. While those are cooling down, take out a big bowl and whip the cream until it is softly done. Stir the yogurt in through the cream.
5. Take your strawberries or other berry of choice and chop it into small pieces. Add this to the cream mixture.
6. Sprinkle the cooled down cream mixture into it and then place into the serving bowls with some dark chocolate on top.

Peppermint and Dark Chocolate Pots

What's inside:

- Peppermint essence (2 drops)
- Stevia (2 drops)
- Egg yolks (4)
- Melted dark chocolate (3 oz.)
- Heavy cream (2.5 c.)

How to make:

1. Take out a bowl and combine the peppermint essence, melted chocolate, stevia, cream, and beaten egg yolks together.
2. Prepare these pots by taking out six ramekins and getting them set up with butter.
3. Pour the chocolate mixture evenly into each of the ramekins and then place these into the slow cooker.
4. Carefully pour some hot water into the pot until it gets halfway up these prepared pots.
5. When this is done, add the lid onto the top of the slow cooker and set the temperature level to high.
6. After two hours of cooking, you can take the pots out of the slow cooker and give them time to cool down.
7. Serve with a fresh mint leaf and a bit of whipped cream on the top and enjoy.

Vanilla Custard

What's inside:

- Stevia
- Vanilla (2 tsp.)
- Beaten egg yolks (4)
- Full fat cream (3 c.)

How to make:

1. Take out a bowl and whisk together the stevia, vanilla, egg yolks, and cream together.
2. Pour this mixture into a dish that is heat proof and will fit into the slow cooker. Add this dish into your slow cooker.
3. Pour in enough hot water that it will fit halfway around the sides of that dish, and then add the lid on top.
4. Turn the slow cooker on and let it get to the high setting. After three hours, the dessert is done and you can serve, either hot or cold.

Coconut and Almond Truffle Bake

What's inside:

- Chopped and toasted almonds (25. C.)
- Heavy cream (1 c.)
- Heavy cream (1 c.)
- Vanilla (2 tsp.)
- Cocoa powder (3 Tbsp.)
- Desiccated coconut (1 c.)
- Ground almonds (1 c.)
- Melted dark chocolate (3 oz.)
- Melted butter (3 oz.)

How to make:

1. Bring out a bowl and mix together the vanilla, cocoa powder, coconut, ground almonds, chocolate, and melted butter.
2. Take this mixture and then roll it into some smaller balls.
3. Prepare a heat proof dish and grease it with some butter. Make sure that it fits into the slow cooker.
4. Place the balls into this dish and then place the dish into the slow cooker. Add the lid on top.
5. Turn on the slow cooker to a low temperature and let it cook. After four hours, take the dish out of the slow cooker and let it cool down.
6. Take out a bowl and whip the cream until it is soft and kind of pillowy.
7. Spread this cream over the truffle dish and then sprinkle some of the grated chocolate and toasted almonds on the top. Serve right away.

Peanut Butter Cupcakes

What's inside:

- Toasted and chopped pecans (10)
- Cinnamon (1 tsp.)
- Baking powder (1 tsp.)
- Ground almonds (1 c.)
- Lightly beaten eggs (2)
- Coconut oil (2 Tbsp.)
- Dark chocolate (5 oz.)
- Vanilla (2 tsp.)
- Butter (2 oz.)
- Smooth peanut butter (1 c.)
- Paper cupcake cases (14)

How to make:

1. To start this recipe, melt together the coconut oil and dark chocolate in the microwave. Stir around to combine and then set it aside.
2. Place the butter and the peanut butter in a bowl and then microwave this as well. Do it for just thirty seconds at a time until the butter just starts to melt. Stir together to make these smooth.
3. Add the vanilla to the peanut butter mixture as well. Then take another small bowl out and combine the cinnamon, baking powder, eggs, and ground almonds together.
4. Pour the coconut milk and the chocolate evenly into the 14 paper cases. Spoon half of the almond and egg mixture evenly into the cases over the chocolate, and then press it down.
5. Spoon the peanut butter mixture into the cases on top of the rest, and then finish off with the rest of the egg and almond mixture.
6. Sprinkle on some of the chopped pecans to the top of the cupcakes. Then place these into the slow cooker. You can use a rack if all of these don't fit on well.
7. Place the lid on top of the slow cooker and set the temperature to a high setting. After four hours, take the cakes out of the slow cooker and give them time to cool down.
8. Serve the cupcakes with some whipped cream on top.

Vanilla and Strawberry Cheesecake

What's inside:

Base
- Cinnamon (1 tsp.)
- Vanilla (2 tsp.)
- Desiccated coconut (.5 c.)
- Ground hazelnuts (1 c.)
- Melted butter (2 oz.)

Filling
- Chopped strawberries (8)
- Vanilla (2 tsp.)
- Sour cream (1 c.)
- Beaten eggs (2)
- Cream cheese (2 c.)

How to make:

1. To start this recipe, we need to work on the base first. To do this, take out a bowl and combine together the cinnamon, vanilla, coconut, hazelnuts, and melted butter.
2. Press this base into a heat proof dish that can also fit into your slow cooker.
3. In a big bow, add the vanilla, sour cream, eggs, and cream cheese. Beat with an egg beater until it is thick and combined.
4. Fold the strawberries into this cream cheese mixture and then pour it on top of your base, making sure to spread it out until smooth.
5. Place this baking dish into the slow cooker and then add in enough hot water so that it can come up to the halfway point of the pan.
6. Add a lit to the slow cooker and then set the temperature to a low setting.
7. After six hours, the cheesecake should be slightly wobbly, but done. Take it out of the slow cooker and then let it cool down. Then add to the fridge until cold.
8. Serve with some whipped cream and enjoy.

Macadamia Fudge Truffles

What's inside:

- Lightly beaten egg (1)
- Vanilla (1 tsp.)
- Melted dark chocolate (5 oz.)
- Melted butter (2 oz.)
- Ground almonds (.5 c.)
- Chopped macadamia nuts (1 c.)

How to make:

1. Take out a big bowl and combine together the egg, vanilla, melted chocolate, melted butter, almonds, and macadamia nuts.
2. Take out your slow cooker and then grease the bottom with some butter. Place this mixture into the slow cooker and press it down.
3. Add the lid onto the slow cooker and then turn the temperature onto a low setting.
4. After four hours, take the lid off the slow cooker and give the mixture some time to cool down until warm.
5. Take a teaspoon and then scoop this mixture out of the pot. Roll these into balls until all of the mixture is used up.
6. Add these on a plate and then put into the fridge to harden a bit. Store in the fridge or eat right away.

Bacon and Chocolate Cupcakes

What's inside:

- Vanilla (1 tsp.)
- Greek yogurt (.5 c.)
- Beaten eggs (2)
- Baking powder (1 tsp.)
- Ground hazelnuts (1 c.)
- Melted dark chocolate (5 oz.)
- Streaky bacon (5 slices)
- Paper cupcake cases (10)

How to make:

1. Take out a bowl and add the melted chocolate with the fried bacon pieces and set it to the side.
2. In a second bowl, mix together the salt, vanilla, yogurt, eggs, baking powder, and ground hazelnuts.
3. Spoon this hazelnut mixture into the cupcake cases and then add the chocolate and bacon mixture to the top of this.
4. Add the cupcake cases to the slow cooker, being careful not to spill, and then add the lid on top. Make sure to set it to the high temperature setting.
5. After three hours, you can take the cupcakes out of the slow cooker and give them time to cool down before serving with some whipped cream.

Coconut Squares with Blueberry Glaze

What's inside:

- Frozen berries (1 c.)
- Vanilla (2 tsp.)
- Baking powder (.5 tsp.)
- Beaten egg (1)
- Cream cheese (3 oz.)
- Melted butter (1 oz.)
- Desiccated coconut (2 c.)

How to make:

1. To start this recipe, bring out a big bowl and beat together the vanilla, baking powder, egg, cream cheese, butter, and coconut. Beat until it is smooth.
2. Bring out a dish that is heat proof and can fit in the slow cooker. Grease it with some butter.
3. Spread your coconut mixture into the bottom of the dish. Add the blueberries to a bowl and then defrost in the microwave until they start to look like a thick sauce.
4. Spread this mixture on top of your coconut mixture. Add the dish to the slow cooker and then add enough hot water to the pot to go halfway up the pan.
5. Add the lid to the slow cooker and then turn the temperature to a high setting.
6. After three hours, take the dish out of the pot and give it time to cool down. Once these are cooled down, you can slice into small squares and serve.

Conclusion

Thank for making it through to the end of Keto Diet Slow Cooker Cookbook 2020, let's hope it was informative and able to provide you with all of the tools you need to achieve your goals whatever they may be.

The next step is to start your journey with the ketogenic diet. This guidebook has all the tools that you need to be successful with the ketogenic diet. Whether you are trying to learn more about this diet plan, you want to be able to improve your health, or you are looking for some great recipes and a meal plan to make the diet plan easier, this guidebook has the information that you need to get started!

Finally, if you found this book useful in any way, a review on Amazon is always appreciated!

Description

The ketogenic diet stands the test of time, and beats out all of the competition in the diet and fitness world. Time and time again, we see that there are a ton of great benefits that come with this diet plan, and anyone is able to see results in just a few weeks when they get started. But where are you supposed to start when it comes to the ketogenic diet? What steps do you need to take, what foods should you eat, and what tips should you follow to make sure that you actually follow the ketogenic diet and see the results that you want?

This guidebook is going to take some time to look at the ketogenic diet and all that it has to offer. The ketogenic diet is taking the world by storm, but the best way to ensure that it actually works for you is to do your research and learn more about how to use it. Luckily, this diet plan is easy, and you will catch on and see amazing weight loss benefits in no time.

What's even better is that we will learn exactly how to use the crock pot to make some delicious meals with this plan. While many people want to join the ketogenic diet to see weight loss and health benefits many don't have hours to spend in the kitchen making these delicious meals. The crockpot can help you make many great ketogenic diet meals that are ready for you when you come home.

Some of the different topics that we will take a look at when it comes to the ketogenic diet includes:

1. The basics of the ketogenic diet
2. The health benefits of going on the ketogenic diet
3. The best foods to eat to remain keto
4. Some of the precautions that you should take when you get started on the ketogenic diet.
5. The benefits of working with the slow cooker.
6. Tips to using the slow cooker to make the ketogenic diet easier.
7. An easy meal plan that can help you get the most out of the ketogenic diet in just three weeks.
8. Some tasty recipes for breakfast, lunch, dinner, sides, and desserts.

When you are ready to learn more about the ketogenic diet and how it can improve your life, and you want to see results quickly, make sure to check out this guidebook to help you get started.

CPSIA information can be obtained
at www.ICGtesting.com
Printed in the USA
BVHW012058220920
589430BV00013B/658

9 781951 764388